DAVID O. MCKAY LIBRARY

D0583538

NOV 2 2 2002

WITHDRAWN

MAR 0 8 2023

DAVID O. McKAY LIBRARY
BYU-IDAHO

PROPERTY OF:
DAVID O. McKAY LIBRARY
BYU-IDAHO
REXBURG ID 83460-0405

Basic Science, Refraction, and Pathology

THE REQUISITES IN OPHTHALMOLOGY

SERIES EDITOR   **Jay H. Krachmer, MD**
Professor and Chairman
Department of Ophthalmology
University of Minnesota Medical School
Minneapolis, Minnesota

OTHER VOLUMES IN THE REQUISITES IN
OPHTHALMOLOGY SERIES

Anterior Segment

Glaucoma

Neuro-Ophthalmology

Oculoplastic Surgery

Pediatric Ophthalmology and Strabismus

Retina, Choroid, and Vitreous

Visit our website at **www.mosby.com**

Basic Science, Refraction, and Pathology

THE REQUISITES
IN OPHTHALMOLOGY

MORTON E. SMITH, M.D.
Professor Emeritus of Ophthalmology and Pathology
Departments of Ophthalmology and Pathology;
Associate Dean Emeritus
Department of Ophthalmology
Washington University School of Medicine
St. Louis, Missouri

MARILYN C. KINCAID, M.D.
Formerly, Clinical Professor of Opthalmology and Pathology
Departments of Ophthalmology and Pathology
St. Louis University School of Medicine
St. Louis, Missouri

CONSTANCE E. WEST, M.D.
Director, Pediatric Ophthalmology
Abrahamson Pediatric Eye Institute
Children's Hospital Medical Center
Cincinnati, Ohio

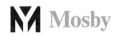 Mosby

An Imprint of Elsevier Science

St. Louis   London   Philadelphia   Sydney   Toronto

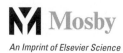

An Imprint of Elsevier Science

11830 Westline Industrial Drive
St. Louis, Missouri 63146

Copyright © 2002 by Mosby, Inc.
An imprint of Elsevier Science

No part of this publication may be reproduced, stored in a retrieval system, or transmitted in any form or by any means, electronic, mechanical, photocopying, recording, or otherwise, without prior permission of the publisher (Mosby Inc., 11830 Westline Industrial Drive, St. Louis, Missouri 63146).

Notice

Ophthalmology is an ever-changing field. Standard safety precautions must be followed, but as new research and clinical experience broaden our knowledge, changes in treatment and drug therapy may become necessary or appropriate. Readers are advised to check the most current product information provided by the manufacturer of each drug to be administered to verify the recommended dose, the method and duration of administration, and contraindications. It is the responsibility of the treating physician, relying on experience and knowledge of the patient, to determine dosages and the best treatment for each individual patient. Neither the Publisher nor the author assume any liability for any injury and/or damage to persons or property arising form this publication.

THE PUBLISHER

ISBN 0-323-00236-6

Acquisitions Editor: Natasha Andjelkovic
Senior Managing Editor: Kathryn Falk
Publishing Services Manager: Patricia Tannian
Project Manager: Melissa Lastarria
Book Design Manager: Gail Morey Hudson

GW/KPT

Printed in the United States of America.

Last digit is the print number: 9   8   7   6   5   4   3   2   1

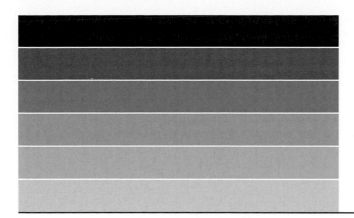

Preface

When my friend and colleague, Dr. Jay Krachmer, asked me to write a chapter on ophthalmic pathology for this volume in his series, *The Requisites in Ophthalmology*, my initial reaction was "Why ? . . . several excellent texts and chapters already exist." He then explained that the *Requisites* fill a void. Where does the ophthalmologist, basic science researcher, or anatomic pathologist go when she or he wants an instant refresher course on the key features of the pathology of specific disease entities? And so the final chapter of *The Requisites in Ophthalmology: Basic Science, Refraction, and Pathology* does not pretend to replace in any way the excellent textbooks that already exist. This chapter assumes that the reader has already had exposure to a basic science course in ophthalmology, a refraction course, and an ophthalmic pathology course. I hope that this chapter fills the aforementioned void.

I was confident in handling the section on ophthalmic pathology, but I had to cry for help with the writing of the sections on basic science and refraction. I am fortunate that the best persons to handle those two sections agreed to come to my rescue. Dr. Marilyn Kincaid has done an outstanding job on Basic Science and Dr. Connie West has done the same exemplary job on Refraction. Dr. Kincaid centers on the general anatomy of each eye segment and its corresponding physiology through various color and black-and-white illustrations. Dr. West offers a comprehensive section on refraction where diagrams and illustrations display how the different components of the retinal image is produced by the eye.

Morton E. Smith, MD
Professor Emeritus
Associate Dean Emeritus
Washington University in St. Louis

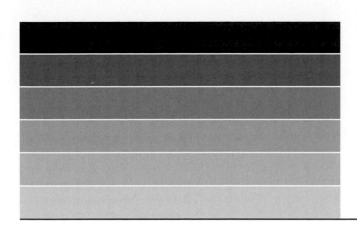

Illustration Acknowledgments

The editor acknowledges Prism Press for permission to use illustrations borrowed from the following publication:

Guyton DL, et al: *Ophthalmic Optics and Clinical Refraction*, 1999, Prism Press.

Mosby Figure	Prism Press page number
11-2, 11-3, 11-4	page 1
11-5, 11-6	page 2
11-7, 11-8	page 11
11-9	page 17
11-10, 11-11	page 13
11-12, 11-13	page 15
11-14, 11-15	page 18
11-16	page 19
11-19	page 14, *top*
12-1	page 20, *top*
12-3, 12-4	page 21
13-1, 13-2	page 22
13-3, 13-5	page 24
13-6	page 25, *middle*
14-16	page 31, *middle*
15-1, 15-2, 15-5 A-C	page 3
15-4	page 4, *top*
15-6	page 6, *top*
16-2, 16-3, 16-4	page 8
18-1, 18-2	page 10, *middle*
18-3	page 32, *middle*
18-4	page 33

Contents

Basic Science, Refraction, and Pathology

THE REQUISITES IN OPHTHALMOLOGY

BASIC SCIENCE

MARILYN C. KINCAID

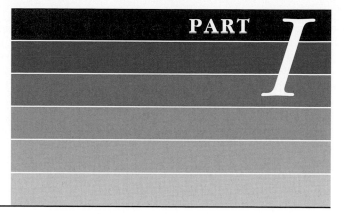

PART *I*

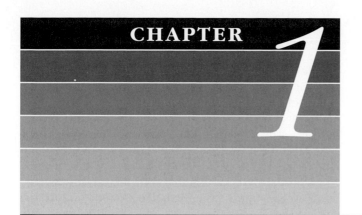

Why Study Basic Science?

Ophthalmology, whether we like it or not, has become more and more technical. A stroll through the exhibitors' section at the annual American Academy of Ophthalmology meeting provides ample evidence of this phenomenon. One can buy the latest gadget for the latest method of microscopic surgery; the only problem is that it will become obsolete the following year. Both medications and surgical procedures are being modified in such a way that outcomes—expected and demanded—are ever more precise. Therefore it is reasonable at the outset to ask, "Why study basic science? How can this material be useful in the day-to-day practice of ophthalmology?"

SERIES OF PROBLEMS TO BE SOLVED

If ocular anatomy, physiology, and biochemistry are simply learned for some sort of expediency, to satisfy some requirement, or to pass some examination, then the answer is simple: there is little use. However, basic science can be understood as the study of problems to be solved. The eye is a wonderful place to consider such a study. Not only are the ocular tissues uniquely suited to their function, but the eye is also easily accessible; we can examine it readily and observe phenomena directly. Study of these tissues and their function provides insight into both normal and abnormal processes.

What is the function of the eye? The eye receives and processes light. We see because information given off in the visible wavelengths of light are received and processed by the eye, then submitted in turn to the brain for further analysis and interpretation. How is this function accomplished? How do the ocular structures allow sight to happen? The purpose of this text is to help understand these phenomena. In so doing, it is possible to understand more fully how things can go wrong, resulting in disease.

TRANSPARENT BUT LIVING MEDIA

At the outset, the most striking thing about the eye is the transparency of certain tissues. As ophthalmologists, we routinely take advantage of this transparency as we examine the eye. We can hear the heart and we can palpate the liver, but we can examine the eye directly through various instruments. Magnification is often all that is needed for examination; for other parts of the examination, we use prisms and mirrors.

However, additional sophisticated techniques for examining the eye and orbit are becoming increasingly routine. Computed tomographic scans, magnetic resonance imaging, and ultrasound scanning and biomicroscopy are all diagnostic methods developed in the past few decades. We often use these techniques to complement our physical examination. They allow us to visualize tissues not otherwise accessible. Other techniques such as fluorescein angiography and psychophysical examinations such as electroretinography allow visualization of dynamic functions of the eye. Knowledge of the relevant anatomy and physiology makes these techniques even more useful. Moreover, these techniques themselves have helped further our understanding of physiologic as well as pathologic ocular function.

INFORMATION GATHERING

The eye is part of the central nervous system. More than half of the cranial nerves (specifically nerves II through VIII) impact the eye in one way or another. The optic nerve is in reality a tract of the brain, and retinal architecture is reminiscent of that of the cerebral cortex. Complex neuronal interactions modulate the information gleaned by the photoreceptors even before it is passed on to the occipital lobe of the cortex. Indeed, Dowling had it right when he considered the eye as "an approachable part of the brain."

THREE INTERRELATED DISCIPLINES

In this section, we will explore the structure and function of the normal eye. This is necessarily brief—the merest introduction. The purpose is to provide a basis for further understanding of normal and abnormal phenomena of the eye, so that additional reading becomes more comprehensible. We stress concepts and mechanisms in the belief that understanding, rather than rote memorization, is the key to further learning, as well as to enjoyment of the learning process.

The suggested readings at the end of this chapter include several relevant textbooks for further, deeper exploration of these concepts. Many of the individual chapters in these reference books also pertain to the other chapters in this text.

The three interrelated disciplines are anatomy, physiology, and biochemistry. "Interrelated" is the key concept; indeed it is difficult to compartmentalize these disciplines, as should become more obvious as we proceed.

For all of these disciplines, we can consider a series of "problems" to be "solved" by the organism. But first, we should consider some general principles.

Anatomy and Histology

Anatomy is the study of structure. Gross anatomy and microscopic anatomy (histology) both provide descriptions of how an organism is put together. Furthermore, the arrangement of these structures is not random. Embryology, the study of prenatal development, helps us understand how the tissue or organism came to be that way.

Structure related to function Tissues and the cells within them have specific functions within the organism, and therefore the tissue structures reflect those particular needs. A photoreceptor cell does not look like a liver cell, for example, nor are all the same biochemical and physiologic processes active in each. The "average cell" does not exist, but there are certain common denominators (Fig. 1-1).

The cell is enclosed by a unit membrane, also called a plasma membrane, a structure about 7.5 nm thick. This forms the outer boundary (Fig. 1-2). It consists of a double layer of lipids, usually phospholipids, oriented so that the chains, which are hydrophobic, are toward the center of the membrane, and the "heads" of the lipid molecules, which are hydrophilic, or water-miscible, are outward. There are regional modifications of this structure, however. Proteins can bind either on the outer surface of the cell or on the inner surface within the cell. Some proteins are mounted within the unit membrane itself, so that part of the molecule extends outside the cell and part extends into the cytoplasm. The regions of the proteins that span the plasma membranes are usually αhelixes, while the loops inside or outside the cell may have other tertiary structures. One example of such a molecule is rhodopsin, which crosses the unit membrane seven times. Ion channels, such as those for calcium and sodium ions, also span the plasma membrane several times. These proteins act as gatekeepers, allowing or prohibiting crossing by certain small molecules, depending on conditions. To do this, these proteins tend to undergo conformational changes.

Virtually all living cells have a nucleus. (Exceptions include lens fibers and circulating red blood cells, which have lost their nuclei.) The nucleus of the cell is basophilic and appears purple on routine (hematoxylin and eosin) staining, reflecting the high nucleic acid content. Within the nucleus are the chromosomes, which contain deoxyribonucleic acid (DNA), the master "blueprint" that directs the structure of proteins in the cell. Individual chromosomes cannot be visualized in the nondividing cell. The nucleus is also surrounded by a unit membrane, and it too has focal modifications.

The cytoplasm of many cells is eosinophilic, appearing blandly pink on routine staining. This blandness hides the fact that the cytoplasm is highly organized; this organization is not fully appreciated without the higher magnification afforded by electron microscopy. There are many organelles of the cell; for the cell they are the counterparts of organs in a living thing (see Fig. 1-1).

One of the most important of these organelles is the mitochondrion. Mitochondria may have originally been a type of bacteria, and thus parasitic in the cell; they are now indispensable to cellular function. They have their own DNA, which codes for many of the enzymes essential for energy storage. Ultrastructurally they appear as oval or sinuous structures with a double membrane. The inner membrane is much greater in surface area than the outer; thus the inner membrane is infolded numerous times, forming cristae. The specific configuration of the mitochondria and their cristae varies from cell to cell, but in general, cells that have many mitochondria are active in aerobic, or oxygen-requiring, metabolism.

Another organelle is endoplasmic reticulum, a long, convoluted unit membrane within the cell. Rough endo-

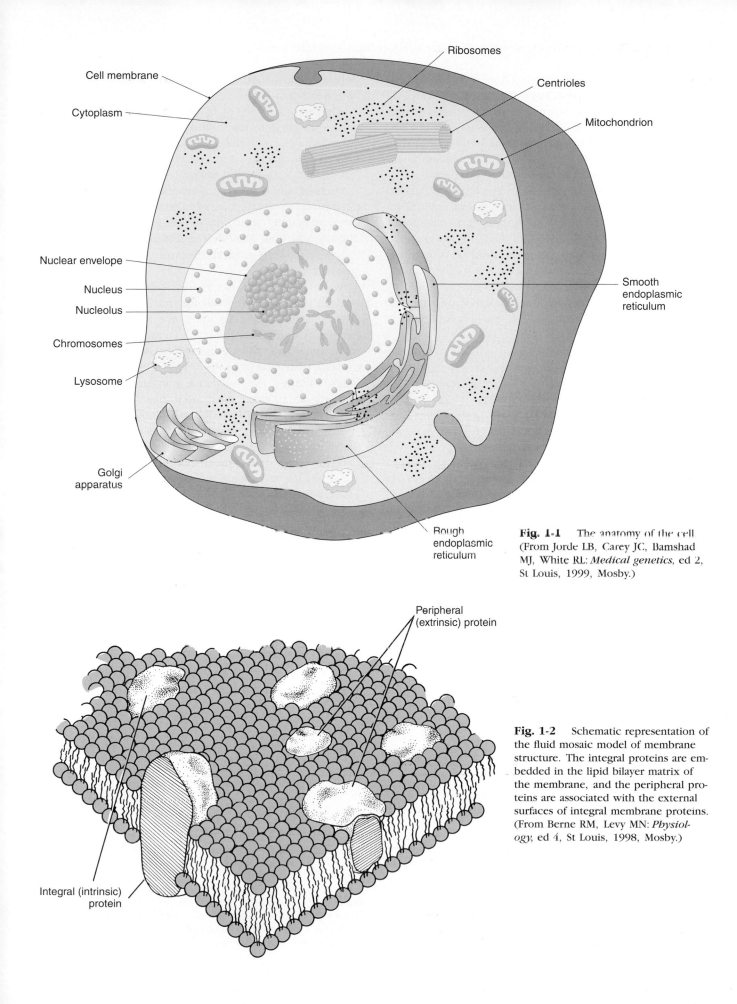

Cell membrane

Cytoplasm

Ribosomes

Centrioles

Mitochondrion

Nuclear envelope

Nucleus

Nucleolus

Chromosomes

Lysosome

Smooth endoplasmic reticulum

Golgi apparatus

Rough endoplasmic reticulum

Fig. 1-1 The anatomy of the cell. (From Jorde LB, Carey JC, Bamshad MJ, White RL: *Medical genetics*, ed 2, St Louis, 1999, Mosby.)

Peripheral (extrinsic) protein

Integral (intrinsic) protein

Fig. 1-2 Schematic representation of the fluid mosaic model of membrane structure. The integral proteins are embedded in the lipid bilayer matrix of the membrane, and the peripheral proteins are associated with the external surfaces of integral membrane proteins. (From Berne RM, Levy MN: *Physiology*, ed 4, St Louis, 1998, Mosby.)

plasmic reticulum, which is reticulum with ribosomes attached, is the site of protein synthesis. By electron microscopy, the ribosomes appear as dark dots lining the membrane. Proteins and other molecules synthesized for export are packaged and discharged out of the cell by the Golgi apparatus, a series of concentric unit membranes adjacent to areas of rough endoplasmic reticulum.

Cells have a disposal mechanism, the lysosome. Lysosomes are spherical, unit-membrane bound organelles that contain digestive enzymes. Depending on metabolic activity, these may be large or small. Over the years, cells accumulate waste products, indigestible end-products of metabolism. These accumulate within lysosomes as a variably electron-dense material called lipofuscin. Certain cells contain melanin, which is synthesized and retained within melanosomes.

Physiology

Physiology can be thought of as dynamic anatomy. Now that we have the structure, how does it work? What processes make it do what it does? Some functions are "vegetative," requisite for life itself. Other functions occur as reactions to stimuli.

Transport   Important aspects of physiology are the structure and function of membranes. Membranes act as semipermeable barriers between nucleus and cytoplasm,

between cytosol and the cytoplasmic organelles, and between cell and cell.

The body is a series of compartments. These compartments include the blood plasma, the extracellular compartment, and the intracellular space. Substances must be able to get from one compartment to another, but only in a controlled fashion.

Permeability is relative. The cell plasma membrane is permeable to water, but whether it is permeable to a given molecule or an ion depends on its size, shape, charge, and lipid solubility. Substances may get across the membrane by several mechanisms, either active or passive.

Passive transport occurs by diffusion and simply means that a substance will migrate across from where its concentration is greater to where it is less (Fig. 1-3). Eventually equilibrium is reached, where the net movement toward one side of the membrane is the same as the movement to the opposite side. This equilibrium remains dynamic; the substance continues to cross from one side to another, even after the relative concentrations on the two sides have come into balance.

If a membrane is permeable to water, but not to a given solute, then water will cross over toward the side with the solute. This movement increases the amount of water on the side with the solute compared with the other side. This phenomenon is called osmosis. The os-

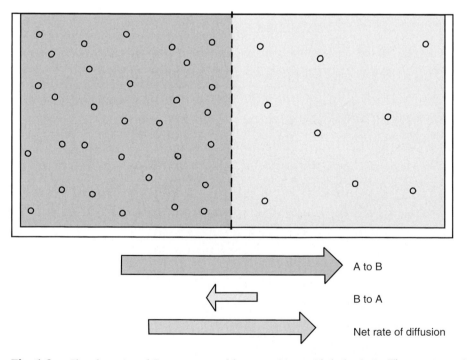

Fig. 1-3   Chambers A and B are separated by a partition with holes in it. The concentration of molecules in chamber A is much greater than that in chamber B. For this reason, the rate of diffusion of molecules from A to B is much greater than that from B to A. There is thus a net flux of molecules from A to B. (From Berne RM, Levy MN: *Physiology*, ed 4, St Louis, 1998, Mosby.)

motic pressure is the pressure necessary to prevent the water from moving.

Another passive process is ultrafiltration. This occurs when there is either hydrostatic pressure or an osmotic gradient across the membrane. In the body, ultrafiltration is one of the processes involved in the production of fluids derived from blood. In the eye, this includes aqueous fluid formation.

There are channels in the plasma membrane, as noted above. These channels allow entry or exit of specific solutes, and may be always open or only be open under specific conditions. Some of these channels simply facilitate diffusion, allowing entry of a bulky molecule such as glucose.

Other channels transport substances against gradient, a process called active transport, which requires energy. This energy is nearly always derived from hydrolysis of adenosine triphosphate (ATP). An example is the sodium-potassium pump, which exchanges sodium for potassium within the cell.

Biochemistry

Biochemistry underpins biologic processes. Structure and function are rooted in chemical reactions that allow buildup and breakdown of complex molecules to permit the functions of life itself. How does the cell handle these myriad essential reactions?

In aggregate, the biochemical reactions of the cell are collectively called metabolism. Metabolism consists of anabolism, the building up of molecules, and catabolism, the breaking down of molecules.

Biochemical reactions are highly efficient. That is, virtually all of a given substrate, or starting molecule, is converted to product. The enzymes that catalyze the reactions are specifically contoured to expedite the biochemical reactions.

Heat dissipation and energy conservation   Anyone who has poured lye down the sink drain recognizes that this chemical reaction, like so many catabolic processes, generates heat. In the open air, this heat quickly dissipates. However, within the cell, heat accumulation is a disaster; it wastes energy and can cause cell death. It is essential to harness this energy for other tasks. Therefore, the cell's problems are to retain energy in a form that can be stored for later use and to minimize lethal heat buildup. In the living organism, this energy conversion results in a remarkably constant internal temperature. The diurnal temperature variation in a human is less than 1° C, despite the furious activity of billions of cells.

The energy is encapsulated in the form of ATP. There are other similar molecules, but ATP is the most common. Energy is then consumed when ATP is subsequently cleaved to form adenosine diphosphate (ADP) and an inorganic phosphate ion.

Anabolism   Anabolism is literally the process of building up. More complex molecules are made up of simpler subunits. For example, proteins are made up of amino acids, fats of fatty acids, complex carbohydrates of monosaccharides, and nucleic acids of purines and pyrimidines, as well as specific monosaccharides. Some of these building blocks are also synthesized in the cell, whereas others must be "imported," absorbed through foodstuffs. This synthesis generally requires energy. Also, some of the enzymes involved in metabolism require various mineral ions, such as calcium, magnesium, and the like or vitamins such as folic acid or niacin.

Catabolism   Catabolism is the process of tearing down. One example of catabolism is digestion; food taken in is broken down into usable components in the stomach, intestine, and liver. This breakdown generally involves the release of energy, which is retrieved and stored as ATP and other similar molecules.

MAJOR POINTS

There is no such thing as an "average" cell. Cell structure is related to its function, and some metabolic pathways are active only in certain cells.

The cell membrane is a double layer of lipids with numerous modifications to allow transit of specific molecules, such as glucose, into and out of the cell under controlled conditions.

Nearly all cells have a nucleus. The cell nucleus contains DNA, the genetic master plan of the organism.

Mitochondria are cytoplasmic organelles that provide cell energy via oxidative phosphorylation. This energy is stored mainly in the form of ATP.

Lysosomes, intracytoplasmic membrane bound structures that contain digestive enzymes, are the cell disposal mechanism for metabolic end-products. Indigestible end-products, such as lipofuscin, accumulate with age within them.

Transport of substances across membranes can be active or passive. Passive processes include osmosis, ultrafiltration, and facilitated transport. Active transport occurs against gradient, via an enzyme pump, and requires energy in the form of ATP.

Many proteins are enzymes that act as highly efficient catalysts for the many chemical reactions that comprise metabolism.

Anabolism, or "building up," is the synthesis of complex product from simpler substrate. This requires energy.

Catabolism is the breakdown of more complex molecules to simpler ones. This process usually allows the release of energy, which is captured and stored as ATP or similar molecules.

SUGGESTED READINGS

Dowling JE: *The retina: an approachable part of the brain,* Cambridge, Mass, 1987, Belknap Press of Harvard University.

Harding JJ, editor: *Biochemistry of the eye,* London, 1997, Chapman & Hall.

Hart WM Jr: *Adler's physiology of the eye,* ed 9, St Louis, 1992, Mosby.

Hogan MA, Alvarado J, Weddell J: *Histology of the human eye,* Philadelphia, 1971, WB Saunders.

Kuwabara T: The eye. In Weiss L, editor, *Histology: cell and tissue biology,* ed 5, pp 1134-1176, New York, 1983, Elsevier Science.

Rodieck RW: *The first steps in seeing,* Sunderland, Mass, 1998, Sinauer Associates.

Spencer WH, editor: *Ophthalmic pathology: an atlas and textbook,* ed 4, Philadelphia, 1998, WB Saunders.

CHAPTER 2

Genetics and Embryology: How It All Begins

How did the eye come to have the structure it has? What processes take place before fertilization and during development? Genetics and embryology help to explain how the structure and function of the mature eye came to be.

Understanding genetics has become increasingly indispensable to comprehending disease, as more and more diseases are found to have a genetic component. Also, gene therapy, once the stuff of science fiction, increasingly appears to offer hope for otherwise untreatable disease.

Embryology helps to explain some of the "whys" of structure. Anatomic findings make more sense when considered along with the cell migration and specialization that occurs during development of the organism.

GENETICS

Genetics is the study of heredity. In recent years there has been a veritable explosion of knowledge concerning modes of inheritance, gene structure and product, and the complex interactions of genetics and environment.

Genes and Chromosomes

It all begins with the union of an egg and a sperm. Indeed, it begins long before that. A baby is born with the cellular antecedents of its own eggs or sperm or, in other words, the beginnings of its own descendants.

Living things have a characteristic number of chromosomes; the number differs for different organisms. For humans, this number is 46, of which 44 are autosomes, 22 matched pairs. One of each pair comes from the father and one from the mother. The autosomes are, by convention, numbered by size, so that chromosome pair number 1 is the largest, and those pairs numbered 20 through 22 are the smallest. In addition, humans have two sex chromosomes. In females there are two X chromosomes, whereas males have an X and a Y chromosome. They are called X and Y because of their shape, and the X chromosome is much larger than the Y.

Chromosomes can now be identified individually by characteristic staining bands (explained more fully in the following), although in the past, similar-sized chromosomes could not be distinguished reliably. Thus chromosomes were classified into 7 groups according to size. Chromosomes 1 through 3, the largest, were part of the A group, and so forth. For example, trisomy 18, in which there are three chromosomes 18, is sometimes referred to in the older literature as trisomy E, because chromosome 18, along with 16 and 17, which are morphologically similar, comprise the E group.

Chromosomes are made up of deoxyribonucleic acid (DNA), the master blueprint for heredity. (With the exception of certain viruses, all organisms have DNA, which contains the genetic information for that individual. Some viruses, called *retroviruses*, have ribonucleic acid [RNA] instead of DNA as the genomic nucleic acid. These viruses also encode one or more proteins known as *reverse transcriptases*, which transcribe DNA from

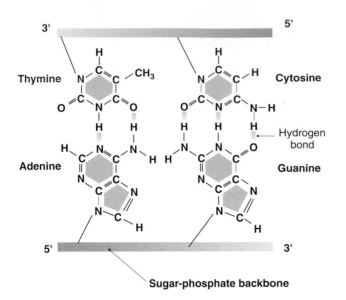

Fig. 2-1   Chemical structure of the four bases, showing hydrogen bonds between base pairs. Three hydrogen bonds are formed between cytosine-guanine pairs, and two bonds are formed between adenine-thymine pairs. (From Jorde LB, Carey JC, Bamshad MJ, White RL *Medical genetics,* ed. 2, St. Louis, 1999, Mosby.)

their genomic RNA.) Each chain of the DNA molecule is a long polymer made up of four possible subunits. Each subunit, called a nucleotide, consists of deoxyribose (the 5-carbon sugar, ribose, missing one oxygen atom, hence "deoxy-") coupled to a phosphate group. Attached to each phosphate group is one of four possible compounds: the purines, adenine (A) and guanine (G), or the pyrimidines, cytosine (C) and thymine (T).

Inherent in the DNA molecule is the ability to make exact copies of itself. This ability comes into play each time a cell divides to give rise to two daughter cells, because each cell requires a full complement of the genome. Each of the nucleotides forms hydrogen bonds with another specific nucleotide—adenine to thymine and guanine to cytosine; thus each of the two strands serves as a template for the generation of its complementary strand. The purine molecules are somewhat larger than the pyrimidine molecules, so all base pairs involve one purine and one pyrimidine (Fig. 2-1).

DNA thus forms a double helix, a kind of twisted ladder configuration, with the sugar-phosphate chains forming the backbones and the purines and pyrimidines forming the rungs (Fig. 2-2).

Fig. 2-2   The structure of the DNA double helix. The sugar-phosphate backbone and nitrogenous bases of each individual strand are arranged as shown. The two strands of DNA pair by forming hydrogen bonds between the appropriate bases to form the double helical structure. The separation of individual strands of the DNA molecule allows DNA replication, catalyzed by DNA polymerase. As the new complementary strands of DNA are synthesized, hydrogen bonds are formed between the appropriate nitrogenous bases. (From Yanoff M, Duker JS: *Ophthalmology,* St Louis, 1999, Mosby.)

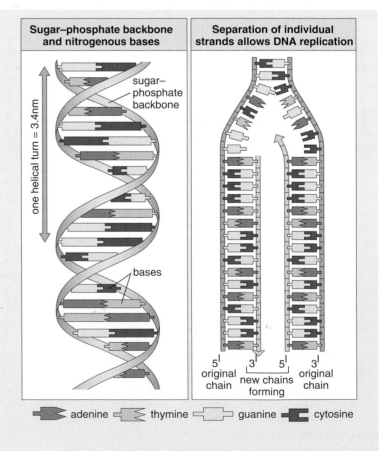

In between cell divisions, DNA serves as the template for generation of RNA, a single-stranded molecule in which ribose replaces deoxyribose and uracil replaces thymine (Fig. 2-3). Generation of RNA is the first step in protein synthesis. There are several types of RNA, but the most important for understanding protein synthesis is messenger RNA (mRNA). Primary messenger RNA is *transcribed* from DNA. The transcribed mRNA is called an *intron*. After transcription, the mRNA is further modified before leaving the nucleus and entering the cytoplasm where protein *translation* takes place; it is now mature mRNA and is called an *exon*.

The human genome consists of about 3.3 billion base pairs. It is estimated that there are up to 100,000 human genes, most of which code for proteins that are a few hundred to a few thousand base pairs long. Thus most of this genetic material does not code for proteins; the precise function of these nontranslated regions is not known.

mRNA is unstable, lasting only a short time in the cytoplasm. This is one way to regulate translation, because only a small amount of protein product is synthesized before the mRNA decomposes.

The genetic code specifies the amino acids that will be linked together to form the protein molecule. A group of three nucleotides is called a *codon;* each amino acid has one or more specific codons. Three of the codons are "stop" codons that terminate translation. Because there are 64 possible three-base combinations of the four nucleotides, but only 20 amino acids specified by the genetic code, the code is obviously redundant. Some amino acids are specified by more than one three-base combination. This is fortunate, because it means that some mutations are silent; in such a case, the original and the mutant codons both specify the same amino acid.

Mitosis

Each chromosome is a linear, nonbranching chain of a specific length. If stretched out, the total amount of DNA in a single human cell would be over 2 meters long. To fit into the cell nucleus, the chromosomes are coiled several times over. Before cell division, the DNA undergoes complete duplication, during the S, or synthesis, phase of the cell cycle.

At the time of cell division, or mitosis, nuclear membrane dissolves and the individual chromosomes separate and become discernible with specific stains (Fig. 2-4). This phase, the beginning of mitosis, is called prophase. At this point the chromosomes can already be seen to have duplicated. Each of the sister chromatids is joined at a single point, the centromere, along the length of the chromosome. The nuclear membrane dissolves, and spindle fibers form from the two centrioles present in the cell. The spindle fibers attach to each centromere.

At metaphase, the point in mitosis when the chromosomes are most condensed, they line up along a single plane. The sister chromatids are pulled apart by the spindle fibers during anaphase, resulting in identical chromosome complements for the two new daughter cells. During telophase, the chromosomes become more elongated and less distinct, and the nuclear membranes again form, as do the cell membranes.

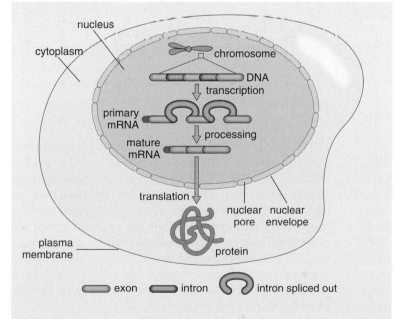

Fig. 2-3   The central dogma of molecular genetics. Transcription of DNA into RNA occurs in the nucleus of the cell, catalyzed by the enzyme RNA polymerase. Mature mRNA is transported to the cytoplasm where translation of the code produces amino acids linked to form a polypeptide chain, and ultimately a mature protein is produced. (From Yanoff M, Duker JS: *Ophthalmology,* St Louis, 1999, Mosby.)

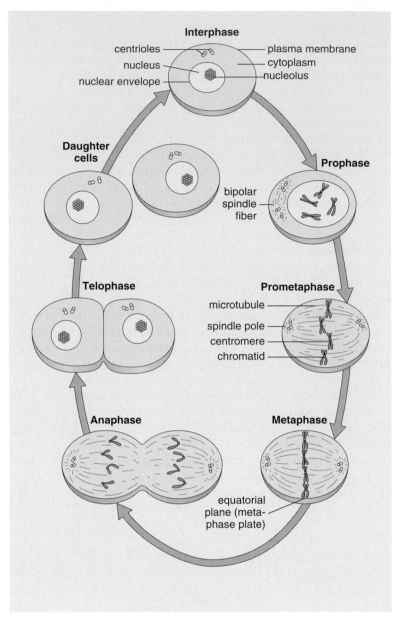

Fig. 2-4   The mitotic cell cycle. During mitosis, the DNA of a diploid cell is replicated, which results in the formation of a tetraploid cell that divides to form two identical diploid daughter cells. (From Yanoff M, Duker JS: *Ophthalmology*, St Louis, 1999, Mosby.)

Chromosomes can be harvested for analysis during late prophase or early metaphase. When appropriately prepared and stained, each chromosome has a specific banding pattern. These bands are numbered according to convention. The shorter arm of each chromosome is designated *p* and the long arm *q*. Bands are numbered starting at the centromere; thus the third band encountered on the short arm of chromosome 1, moving away from the centromere, would be designated 1p3. Subbands are designated with a decimal point after the number of the main band. The number of visible bands can be increased by harvesting the chromosomes somewhat earlier in late prophase, so they are not quite as condensed, and this of course permits higher resolution.

Meiosis and Recombination

The normal chromosome complement present in typical cells is the diploid number. For humans, this number is 46, or 23 pairs. Meiosis is the process whereby eggs and sperm are generated. These germ cells are haploid; they have 23 chromosomes in all, 22 autosomes and a single sex chromosome. When the egg and sperm are united, the result is a new embryo with the diploid number. Because males have an X and a Y chromosome, the resultant sperm may have either one or the other, and it is the specific spermatozoan fertilizing the egg that determines the sex of the baby.

How to account for myriad different human beings? If only whole chromosomes were assorted in the offspring,

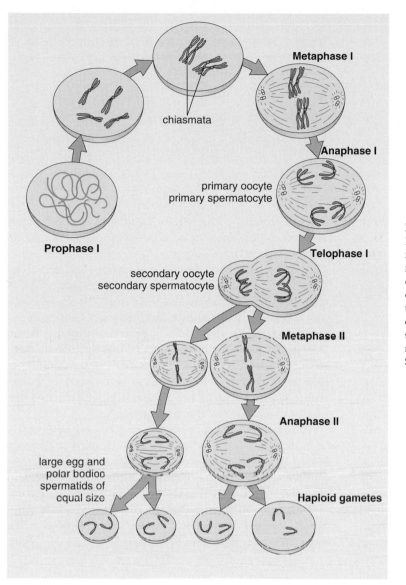

Fig. 2-5   Meiotic cell cycle. During meiosis, the DNA of a diploid cell is replicated, which results in the formation of a tetraploid cell that divides twice to form four haploid cells (gametes). As a consequence of the crossing over and recombination events that occur during the pairing of homologous chromosomes before the first division, the four haploid cells may contain different segments of the original parental chromosomes. For brevity, prophase II and telophase II are not shown. (From Yanoff M, Duker JS. *Ophthalmology*, St Louis, 1999, Mosby.)

there would be relatively little variability from person to person. Yet, except for identical twins, no two individuals have the exact same genetic complement. Meiosis is accomplished in two divisions; during the first division *crossovers* take place.

During the prophase of the first meiotic division, all chromosomes have duplicated, just as they do during mitosis (Fig. 2-5). The difference between mitosis and meiosis is that both chromosomes of each pair become closely associated. The four sister chromatids of each chromosome form a tetrad. Thus there is a tetrad of chromosome 1, a tetrad of chromosome 2, and so on. While the chromosomes are thus aligned, multiple crossovers, or chiasmata, take place along the length of the chromosomes (Fig. 2-6). Only after all these crossovers occur do the chromosomes separate during the anaphase of the first meiotic division.

Crossovers and their frequency help to explain link-

age, a phenomenon of heredity. If two genes are located close to each other on a chromosome, it is unlikely that a crossover will occur between them. The closer together they are, the less likely it is that the two genes will become separated from each other by an intervening crossover. Such genes are said to be linked, and the traits encoded by these two genes will therefore tend to manifest together in the offspring. It is possible, through observation of many individuals as well as through laboratory techniques, to estimate the degree of linkage. Totally random assortment (no linkage, as would occur if the two genes are on different chromosomes) has a linkage score of 1, while complete linkage (if the two genes are in fact identical) has a score of 0. Geneticists use a statistically more powerful method for analyzing the probability of linkage versus random assortment, called the logarithm of the odds ratio, or *lod score*.

Fig. 2-6   Genetic recombination by crossing-over. Two copies of a chromosome are copied by DNA replication. During meiosis, pairing of homologous chromosomes occurs, which enables a crossover between chromosomes to take place. During cell division the recombined chromosomes separate into individual daughter cells. (From Yanoff M, Duker JS: *Ophthalmology,* St Louis, 1999, Mosby.)

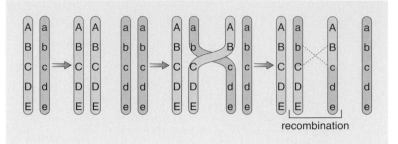

Mendelian Inheritance

Many characteristics are encoded by single genes, and these are inherited according to laws elucidated by Gregor Mendel. Because an individual has two of every autosome, there are two copies of each gene, one copy from the mother and one from the father. These two copies are referred to as *alleles.* If the two alleles are identical, the individual is homozygous for that trait. If they are not, the individual is a heterozygote.

Autosomal dominant traits require a single copy of the gene for the trait to be expressed. Individuals might therefore be homozygous or heterozygous for the trait, but both would appear phenotypically similar. Also, autosomal dominant traits, either traits that are physiologic variants or that are pathologic conditions, are observable and known in a family. Hence, with a disorder such as granular corneal dystrophy, members of a patient's family who also show the abnormal findings can be found. As a general rule (with exceptions!), dominant traits tend to be structural. The risk of inheritance of an autosomal dominant trait is 50%, assuming no other variables (Fig. 2-7).

In contrast, autosomal recessive traits require both copies of the gene to manifest the condition. The patient is typically the first in the genetic line to show the condition, because the heterozygous parents would be unaware that they each carried the recessive trait. Recessive traits are often enzymatic, because in the heterozygous state, enough enzyme is present, albeit in subnormal quantity, to produce adequate normal product. In many conditions for which the enzyme defect is known, it is possible to test for enzyme activity in a heterozygote and demonstrate that it is about half of the normal level. An example is tyrosinase-negative oculocu-

taneous albinism. The risk for an offspring to inherit an autosomal recessive trait from both heterozygous parents is 25% (Fig. 2-7).

A special case is X-linked (sometimes referred to as sex-linked) recessive inheritance. Females have two X chromosomes, but males have only one. Therefore a condition such as Nettleship-Falls ocular albinism tends to affect only males (Fig. 2-7). A female could also be affected, but only if she inherited an X chromosome both from her affected father and from her carrier mother. As with heterozygotes carrying autosomal recessive characteristics, female carriers of X-linked diseases can be identified by assaying for the gene product.

Females are actually mosaics for X-linked traits. Early in embryonic development, one of the two X chromosomes is inactivated in each cell. Thus, on average, in half the cells the active X chromosome is inherited from the mother and in half from the father. There are exceptions to this 50:50 mix, mostly because which X chromosome is inactivated is a random event that follows a bell-shaped distribution curve.

Mitochondrial Genetics

Mitochondria are cellular organelles critical for energy formation. They contain the enzymes of the oxidative phosphorylation pathway; thus they participate in aerobic metabolism and generate adenosine triphosphate (ATP), which can be thought of as the "energy" molecule.

Mitochondria have their own DNA (mtDNA). Rather than being linear, as in higher organisms, it is arranged as a circle, similar to the DNA of bacteria. In addition, the genetic code is somewhat different for this DNA.

Mitochondria are inherited through the maternal line. This makes sense when we remember that the egg has a considerable amount of cytoplasm, whereas the sperm has virtually none, and mitochondria reside in the cytoplasm. Thus mitochondrial diseases may appear to be autosomal dominant, but with mitochondrial disease there can be no father-to-offspring inheritance (Fig. 2-7). Also, the mitochondrial genome is highly conserved, be-

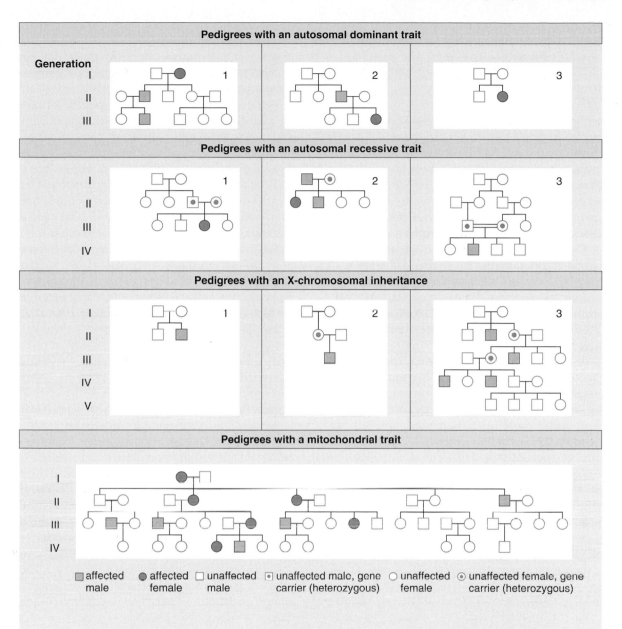

Fig. 2-7   Patterns of inheritance. For pedigrees with an autosomal dominant trait, panel 1 shows inheritance that originates from a previous generation, panel 2 shows segregation that originates in the second generation of this pedigree, and panel 3 shows an apparent "sporadic" case, which is actually a new mutation that arises in the most recent generation—this mutation has a 50% chance of being passed to offspring of the affected individual. For pedigrees with an autosomal recessive trait, panel 1 shows an isolated affected individual in the most recent generation (whose parents are obligatory carriers of the mutant gene responsible for the condition); panel 2 shows a pair of affected siblings whose father is also affected (for the siblings to be affected, the mother must be an obligate carrier of the mutant gene); and panel 3 shows an isolated affected individual in the most recent generation who is a product of consanguineous marriage between two obligate carriers of the mutant gene. For pedigrees with an X-chromosomal trait, panel 1 shows an isolated affected individual whose disease is caused by new mutation in the gene responsible for this condition; panel 2 shows an isolated individual who inherited a mutant copy of the gene from the mother (who is an obligate carrier); and panel 3 shows segregation of an X-linked trait through multi-generation pedigree (50% of the male offspring are affected, and their mothers are obligate carriers of the disease). For pedigrees with a mitochondrial trait, the panel shows a large, multigeneration pedigree—men and women are affected, but only women have affected offspring. (From Yanoff M, Duker JS: *Ophthalmology,* St Louis, 1999, Mosby.)

cause the mtDNA does not participate in nuclear genetic recombinations. A number of mitochondrial diseases affect the eye; Kearns-Sayre syndrome is one example.

Genetic Analysis

Because males have only one X chromosome, it was the first to be mapped in detail with different X-linked diseases and conditions. Subsequently, through use of various marking techniques, genes have been assigned to all the autosomes as well. Many of these have been genes that cause ophthalmic disease.

How can this be done? Linkage studies make assigning genes to specific locations on the chromosomes possible (Fig. 2-8). One can estimate how close a genetic marker is to the gene causing disease by studying families with the inherited disease and different alleles, or structural variants, of the marker gene. In this way, the retinoblastoma gene was found to be closely linked to the gene encoding esterase D, an enzyme whose location was already known.

DNA probes that bind to the gene of interest are a way to refine the mapping assignment and to counsel families with a genetic disease. The area of chromosomal DNA where the probe had bound can be isolated and then treated with one or more restriction endonucleases. Restriction endonucleases are enzymes that cleave DNA at specific, or "restricted," sites. For example, a restriction endonuclease might cut the DNA in the middle of the nucleotide sequence ATTTTA. The result will be a number of DNA fragments of varying size, either beginning with ATT or ending with TTA. These pieces can be separated by electrophoresis. If a person has a mutation that alters one of these sites, for example, turning it into ATTCTA, then cleavage no longer can occur at that site, and the resulting electrophoretic pattern will be different, with one larger piece instead of the two smaller

pieces yielded by the original cleavage site. The variations in the fragments are called restriction fragment length polymorphisms. Because these polymorphisms are also inherited, they also function as markers for the disease gene in question.

Once the gene is mapped to a specific location, it may then be possible to isolate it, sequence it, and identify mutations. Also, genes known to be at the same location on the chromosome can be examined as possible candidates for causing the disease in question. For example, autosomal dominant retinitis pigmentosa was mapped to an area of chromosome 3 where rhodopsin had already been assigned. Analysis of the rhodopsin gene disclosed mutations that caused retinitis pigmentosa.

We must remember that a number of different mutations in the DNA sequence can cause similar phenotypes, or clinical manifestations. Conversely, a single mutation can cause different clinical manifestations, as, for example, in the retinal pigment epithelial pattern dystrophies.

EMBRYOLOGY

How does the eye form? The eye is an extension of the brain, and this is reflected in the development and final morphology of the eye. Contributions from the different embryonic layers are summarized in Table 2-1 and explained more fully in the following text.

A fascinating problem in embryology is the control of the cells during their differentiation. How do cells that start off identical (the first few mitotic divisions in the gamete) begin to express the different specific aspects of their genome to become the varied, highly specialized cells of the organs and tissues of the body? This area of genetics and embryology is still being explored, but certain regulatory genes have been identified, called homeo-

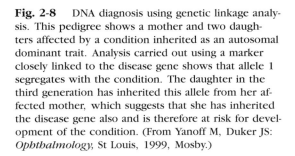

Fig. 2-8 DNA diagnosis using genetic linkage analysis. This pedigree shows a mother and two daughters affected by a condition inherited as an autosomal dominant trait. Analysis carried out using a marker closely linked to the disease gene shows that allele 1 segregates with the condition. The daughter in the third generation has inherited this allele from her affected mother, which suggests that she has inherited the disease gene also and is therefore at risk for development of the condition. (From Yanoff M, Duker JS: *Ophthalmology*, St Louis, 1999, Mosby.)

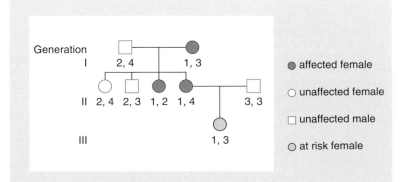

box genes. These function as master genes, because their protein products regulate development. A striking property of these genes is a specific nucleotide sequence that is highly conserved in different homeobox genes

Table 2-1 Origins of ocular structures	
Neuroectoderm	Neuroepithelium
	Sensory retina and optic nerve
Surface ectoderm	Corneal epithelium
	Lids and conjunctiva
	Lens
Neural crest	Corneal and scleral stroma
	Corneal endothelium
	Uveal stroma and melanocytes
	Meninges
Mesoderm	Portions of the sclera
	Ocular blood vessels

from the same species, as well as in species as different as fruit flies and humans. (When scientists list the nucleotide sequences of the different species next to each other, they draw a box around the conserved, or identical, parts of the sequence, hence the name "homeobox.") The protein products of these genes function by binding to DNA, influencing what portions of DNA are transcribed. The conserved region of the gene is the DNA binding site. Alterations in this conserved region prevent proper binding and can lead to specific malformations, such as aniridia, caused by mutations in the *PAX6* homeobox gene.

Neuroectoderm

Early in embryonic life, before 4 weeks of gestation, lateral outpouchings from the telencephalon, the future cerebral cortex, form (Fig. 2-9). These are the optic vesicles, made up of neuroectoderm. Initially their thick-

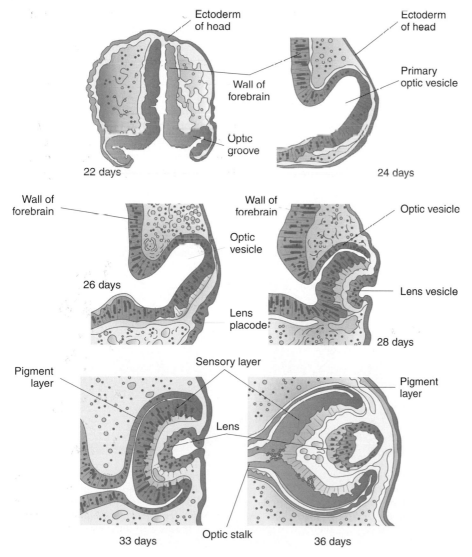

Fig. 2-9   Early development of the human eye. (All drawings are made to the same scale.) (From Carlson BM: *Human embryology and developmental biology,* St Louis, 1994, Mosby.)

ness is a single cell layer, with a basement membrane. The optic vesicle invaginates to form the optic cup. The cup is thus a double cell layer, with the apices of the cells toward each other and the basement membranes away. These two layers will further differentiate to form the neuroepithelial layers of the eye.

Posteriorly, the inner layer proliferates to form the complex sensory retina, whereas the outer layer remains a monolayer, the retinal pigment epithelium (Fig. 2-10). The sensory retina develops into the photoreceptors and other neurons along with their interconnections. The innermost layer of cells, the ganglion cells, send axons back to the brain to form the optic nerve. Vascularization of the retina begins at about the fourth month of gestation. The vessels proceed anteriorly from the optic nerve, reaching the ora serrata at term nasally but not temporally.

Proceeding anteriorly, the portions of the optic cup that will line the ciliary body and iris both remain as monolayers. Overlying the ciliary body, the inner layer remains nonpigmented, the nonpigmented ciliary epithelium, and the outer layer, continuous with retinal pigment epithelium, is the pigmented ciliary epithelium.

In the region of the iris, it is easier to understand the two layers as anterior and posterior, while realizing that they remain inner and outer, respectively. The posterior layer takes on pigmentation, becoming the iris pigment epithelium. The anterior layer partially differentiates into smooth muscle, while remaining partially epithelial and pigmented. The rim of the optic cup is therefore at the pupillary margin. The sphincter muscle surrounding the pupil is composed of migrated neuroectodermal cells also.

Pigmentation of the neuroectoderm takes place very early in embryonic development and is complete by the sixth gestational week. Moreover, it is independent of racial or familial pigmentation (Fig. 2-10). It appears that normal pigmentation is essential for proper development of the macula and also for the proper orientation of the nerve fibers that will cross at the optic chiasm.

Surface Ectoderm

Meanwhile, the surface ectoderm invaginates and pinches off to form the lens vesicle. Thus the cells of the lens are inward and the basement membrane is outward, surrounding the cells—what we understand clinically as the lens capsule. Over the ensuing weeks, the posterior lens cells elongate and gradually lose their nuclei, becoming lens fibers. The anterior lens cells remain as low cuboidal cells just beneath the capsule anteriorly (Fig. 2-11; see also Fig. 2-9).

Surface ectoderm also folds inward to form the eyelid skin and conjunctiva, the conjunctival fornices, the bulbar conjunctiva, and the corneal epithelium. The lids fuse temporarily, later to open shortly before birth.

Neural Crest

Neural crest cells are cells located to either side of the neural tube during early embryogenesis. They are precursors to many different types of cells, including melanocytes and cells of the peripheral nervous system.

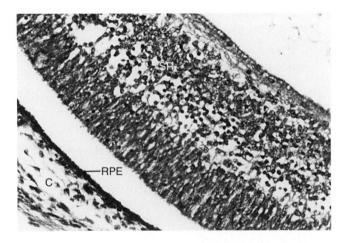

Fig. 2-10   The developing retina *(SR)* and retinal pigment epithelium *(RPE)* in an 11-week embryo. There are two discernible bands of nuclei in the sensory retina. Note that the pigment epithelium is already deeply pigmented, but the subjacent choroid *(C)* is not melanized at this age. Hematoxylin and eosin, ×200. (See color plate.)

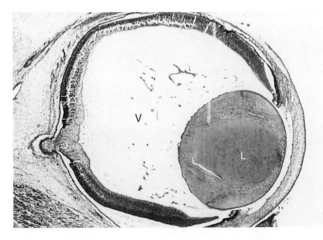

Fig. 2-11   Low power view of an 11-week embryo eye showing the relatively large lens *(L)*. The anterior lens epithelium is discernible beneath the capsule. At the equator, new lens fibers continue to form throughout life. More centrally, the lens fibers have lost their nuclei. Note the blood vessels within the vitreous cavity *(V)*. Hematoxylin and eosin, ×20. (See color plate.)

Within the eye, they form the corneal layers except for the epithelium, the uveal tract stroma, the meninges of the optic nerve, and much of the sclera. Much of what was previously thought to be mesoderm in the eye origi-

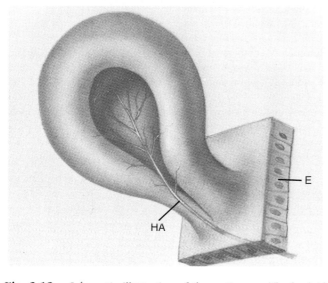

Fig. 2-12 Schematic illustration of the optic cup. The hyaloid artery *(HA)* enters the cup through the inferior embryonic ocular fissure. *E,* Ependymal lining of the diencephalon. (From Apple D, Rabb MF: *Ocular pathology: clinical applications and self-assessment,* ed 5, St Louis, 1998, Mosby.)

nates in fact from the neural crest. Portions of the sclera do receive contributions from mesoderm, and, as elsewhere in the body, the ocular blood vessels are of mesodermal origin.

Pigmentation of the uveal tract melanosomes begins at about the seventh gestational month and continues after birth. The degree of pigmentation is racial and familial, and parallels pigmentation of the skin and hair.

Hyaloid System

The optic cup has an inferonasal defect, the fetal fissure, that extends anteroposteriorly from iris to optic nerve and through which the hyaloid vascular system enters the eye and progresses anteriorly through the vitreous cavity (Fig. 2-12). This vessel branches behind the lens, forming the posterior tunica vasculosa lentis. This system anastomoses with the anterior tunica vasculosa lentis, which arises from the iris and extends across the pupillary space. These vessels are most developed from about 8 to 12 weeks of gestation and then normally regress by the eighth gestational month as the secondary, or adult, vitreous is formed. As the hyaloid system regresses, the fetal fissure closes, starting at about the equator and extending anteriorly and posteriorly. Normally, this closure occurs so perfectly that no scar or defect remains.

MAJOR POINTS

DNA encodes the genetic makeup of the individual. In the nucleus, the DNA is transcribed into RNA, which then exits the nucleus to be translated into protein.

Mitosis is the process of cell division that yields two daughter cells with the identical complement of DNA. Individual chromosomes can only be discerned at this time, because they are so condensed. Between cell divisions, the DNA replicates.

Humans have 46 chromosomes, 44 autosomes, and 2 sex chromosomes (XX in females and XY in males). Each chromosome has a unique banding pattern on special staining; bands are numbered beginning at the centromere. Ocular diseases have been identified and mapped to all the autosomes and the X chromosome.

Meiosis is the process of generating eggs and sperm, which are haploid. During the first of the two meiotic divisions, the chromosome pairs join to form a tetrad and undergo multiple crossovers.

The more closely two genetic loci are on a chromosome, the less likely it is that a crossover will occur between them. Such loci are linked; this linkage can be expressed mathematically and is useful for genetic counseling.

The three major patterns of single-gene inheritance are autosomal dominant, autosomal recessive, and X-linked. Typically, with autosomal recessive inheritance, there is no family history of the trait.

Mitochondrial genes appear to show an autosomal dominant inheritance pattern, but only females pass on the trait to the next generation.

The retina and retinal pigment epithelium, along with the optic nerve, are derived from neuroectoderm; thus they are part of the central nervous system. Continuous with these layers are the epithelial layers of the ciliary body and iris.

The lens of the eye, along with the surface epithelium of cornea and conjunctiva, arises from surface ectoderm. The lens is an "inside out" structure, with the basement membrane forming its outer surface.

Uveal stroma, corneal stroma, corneal endothelium, and much of the sclera are derived from neural crest. The only parts of the eye that come from mesoderm are the blood vessels and portions of the sclera.

Pigmentation in the pigmented neuroepithelial layers is complete by the sixth gestational week; uveal stromal pigmentation begins at the seventh gestational month and is not complete until after birth.

SUGGESTED READINGS

Beebe DC: Homeobox genes and vertebrate eye development, *Invest Ophthalmol Vis Sci* 35:2897-2900, 1994.

Carlson BM: *Human embryology and developmental biology,* St Louis, 1994, Mosby.

Chang TS, Johns DR, Walker D, et al: Ocular clinicopathologic study of the mitochondrial encephalomyopathy overlap syndromes, *Arch Ophthalmol* 111:1254-1262, 1993.

Della NG: Molecular biology in ophthalmology: a review of principles and recent advances, *Arch Ophthalmol* 114:457-463, 1996.

Damji KF, Allingham RR: Molecular genetics is revolutionizing our understanding of ophthalmic disease, *Am J Ophthalmol* 124:530-543, 1997.

Harbour JW: Tumor suppressor genes in ophthalmology, *Surv Ophthalmol* 44:235-246, 1999.

Johns DR: Mitochondrial DNA and disease, *N Engl J Med* 333: 638-644, 1995.

Jorde LB, Carey JC, Bamshad MJ, White RL: *Medical genetics,* ed 2, St Louis, 1999, Mosby.

Kincaid MC: Special laboratory methods for pathological diagnosis of orbital disease, *Int Ophthalmol Clin* 32(3):45-58, 1992.

Mann I: *Development of the human eye,* 3rd ed, New York, 1964, Grune & Stratton.

Puck JM, Willard HF: X inactivation in females with X-linked disease [editorial], *N Engl J Med* 338:325-327, 1998.

Rummelt V, Folberg R, Ionasescu V, et al: Ocular pathology of MELAS syndrome with mitochondrial DNA nucleotide 3243 point mutation, *Ophthalmology* 100:1757-1766, 1993.

Strek W, Strek P, Nowogrodzka-Zagórska M, et al: Hyaloid vessels of the human fetal eye: a scanning electron microscopic study of corrosion casts, *Arch Ophthalmol* 111:1573-1577, 1993.

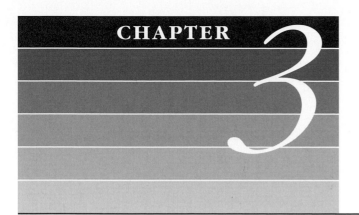

It may seem unnecessary to understand the gross anatomy of the eye if one is not doing dissections. However, many of the landmarks that are observed at dissection also pertain to surgical procedures. One can think of gross dissection as a way to become familiar with these landmarks in an idealized and unhurried setting.

GROSS ANATOMY

The normal adult eye is about 24 mm in diameter. However, the term "adult" is slightly misleading, because the eye attains this size by about the age of 2 to 3 years. At birth, the eye is about 20 mm in diameter. The eyes of small children appear large simply because the eye has attained its adult size long before the facial bones have done so.

The cornea bulges outward because its radius of curvature is smaller than that of the sclera (Fig. 3-1). The limbus varies in width, causing the corneal diameter to be slightly greater horizontally than vertically. However, seen internally, if the iris is removed, the cornea appears circular.

The limbus forms the transition between the transparent cornea and the relatively opaque sclera. Thus clinically it appears somewhat grayish. This transition zone is slightly larger vertically; an advantage for placement of surgical entry wounds. Vertically the limbus measures about 1 mm; horizontally it is about half that. The limbus also forms the transition between the radii of curvature of the sclera and cornea; this makes it a vulnerable spot for ocular rupture with blunt trauma.

If we section the eye into two halves in the sagittal plane, we cut through the macula but find that the optic nerve is in the nasal half. This is to be expected, because the medial walls of the right and left orbits are essentially oriented sagittally and parallel to each other, whereas the lateral walls make a 90° angle. The angle made by the medial and lateral walls of each orbit is thus about half of that, or 45°, and in turn, the angle made by the optic nerve is half of that, or 23° (Fig. 3-2).

The optic nerve posteriorly is about 3 mm in diameter, about twice the diameter of the optic disc. As the nerve fibers exit the eye, they become myelinated. The optic nerve also acquires the meninges. The most obvious meninx grossly is the dura, which becomes continuous with the sclera.

Muscular Landmarks

The movement of each eye is controlled by six extraocular muscles. The four rectus muscles each insert into the globe anterior to the equator. No anatomical landmarks indicate the equator, but for reference, the center of the cornea is the "North Pole."

The spiral of Tillaux refers to the distances of the rectus muscles from the limbus (Table 3-1). Different sources provide somewhat different values for these distances, simply because individual eyes vary. Moreover, the vertical recti insert at an angle, rather than exactly parallel to the limbus, so the limbus-to-muscle distance depends on where the measurement is carried out. The precise measurement is less important than the direction of the spiral. The medial rectus is the muscle closest to the limbus, at a distance of about 5.5 mm. The superior rectus is the farthest, at about 7.7 mm. Spiraling outward, therefore, the muscles in order of distance from the limbus are medial, inferior (about 6.5 mm), lateral (about 7.0 mm), and superior. These muscles insert onto

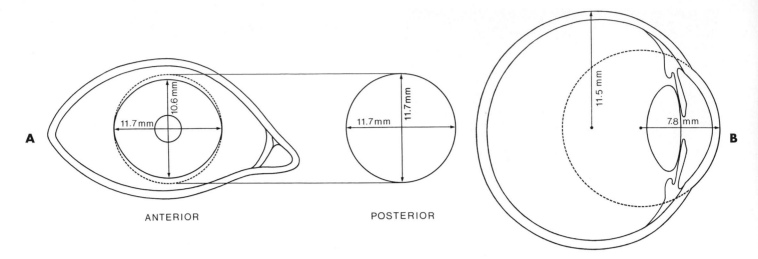

Fig. 3-1 These three diagrams show: **A,** The elliptical shape of the anterior and the round shape of the posterior corneal edges and also the vertical and horizontal diameters of the anterior and the posterior cornea. **B,** The radius of curvature of the cornea and of the sclera. **C,** The corneal height and the central 4 mm of the cornea, which is optically important, and also the comparative thickness of the central and peripheral cornea. (From Hogan MA, Alvarado J, Weddell J: *Histology of the human eye,* Philadelphia, 1971, WB Saunders.)

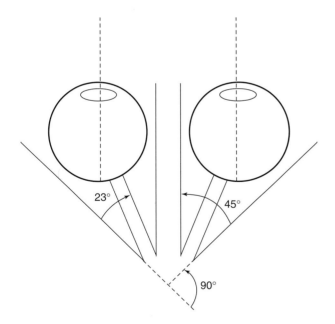

Fig. 3-2 Schematic diagram to show the orientation of the eyes in the orbit. The medial walls are roughly parallel and also parallel to the visual axis. The lateral walls form approximately a 90° angle with each other; thus the two walls of one orbit are at approximately 45°. The optic nerve essentially bisects this angle, so it is about 23° nasal to the fovea.

Table 3-1 Spiral of Tillaux (approximate measurements)

Rectus muscle	Distance from limbus (mm)
Medial	5.5
Inferior	6.5
Lateral	7.0
Superior	7.7

the sclera approximately overlying the ora serrata; thus when one performs rectus recessions, one is suturing over peripheral sensory retina (Fig. 3-3).

The sclera immediately behind the rectus insertions is considerably thinner than it is just anterior to the insertions. If one cuts the muscle attachment as close to the

sclera as possible, the result is a step in the scleral surface (Fig. 3-4).

For dissection purposes, the two oblique muscles are more useful for orienting the globe than the recti. These both insert posterior to the equator. Although functionally the two oblique muscles act in an equal and opposite manner, fortunately for identification purposes, they do differ structurally (Fig. 3-5).

All of the muscles originate at the apex of the orbit except for the inferior oblique, which sweeps laterally and inferiorly from the medial wall of the orbit and underneath the eye. The superior oblique muscle attaches to the globe superiorly, after going through the trochlea, a cartilaginous structure located in the orbit superomedially that acts as a pulley.

The superior oblique muscle, therefore, has the longest tendon of the six extraocular muscles. This makes sense; one would expect that the portion going through the trochlea would be tendinous and nonstretchy. Accordingly, as one inspects the eye, no matter how long

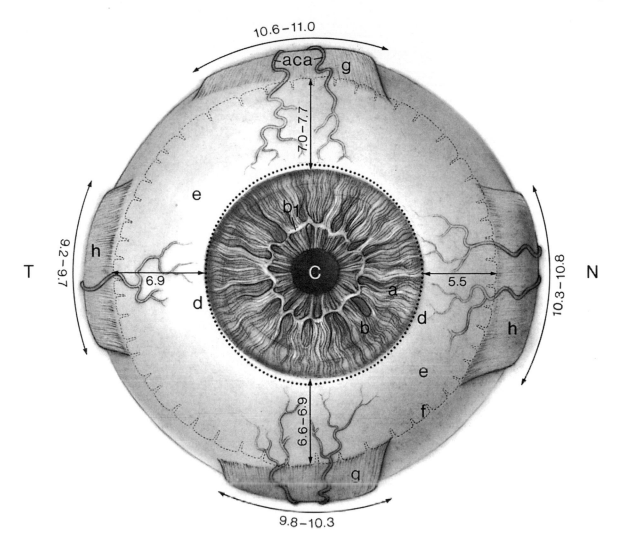

Fig. 3-3   Anterior view of the eyeball showing the cornea *(a)*, iris *(b)*, and pupil *(c)*. The dotted line at *d* indicates the circular nature of the cornea as it would be seen from behind the eye. The sclera is at *e*. The ora serrata is indicated by the dotted line at *f*. The horizontal rectus muscles are at *h* and the vertical ones at *g*. Each rectus muscle has two anterior ciliary arteries except the lateral rectus muscle, which has only one. (From Hogan MA, Alvarado J, Weddell J: *Histology of the human eye,* Philadelphia, 1971, WB Saunders.)

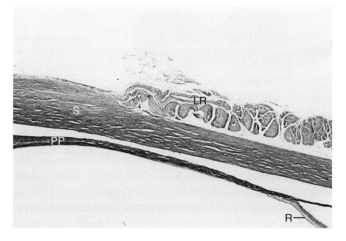

Fig. 3-4   Insertion of the lateral rectus muscle *(LR)* into the sclera *(S)*. Behind the muscle the sclera is considerably thinner. The pars plana *(PP)* is artifactually detached from the sclera. Peripheral retina *(R)* is present posteriorly. Hematoxylin and eosin, ×20. (See color plate.)

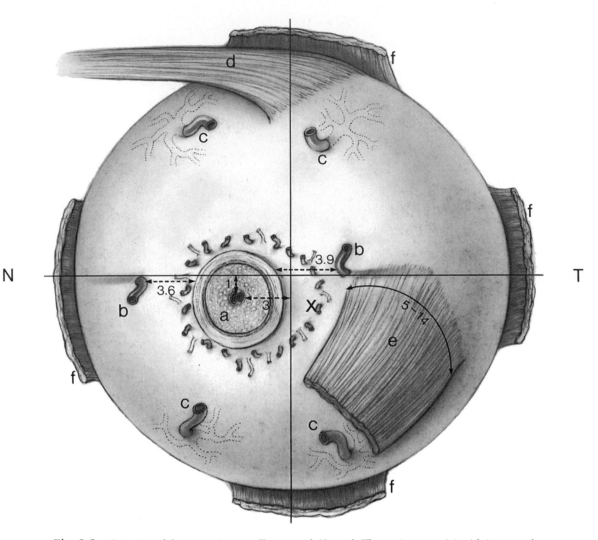

Fig. 3-5   Drawing of the posterior eye. *T,* temporal; *N,* nasal. The optic nerve *(a)* with its central vessels and surrounding meningeal sheaths is seen. Its center is located 3 mm nasal and 1 mm inferior to the posterior pole of the eye. Surrounding it are the short posterior ciliary arteries and nerves. The approximate position of the macula is at *x.* Along the horizontal meridian, which bisects the eye, are the long posterior ciliary arteries and nerves *(b).* The exits of four vortex veins are shown, one for each quadrant *(c).* The curved, oblique insertions of the superior oblique *(d)* and inferior oblique *(e)* muscles are seen. The cut ends of the four rectus muscles are at *f.* (From Hogan MA, Alvarado J, Weddell J: *Histology of the human eye,* Philadelphia, 1971, WB Saunders.)

a remnant is left of the superior oblique, it will appear tendinous. It inserts close to 12 o'clock, at about 11:30 for a right eye and 12:30 for a left.

The inferior oblique muscle, in contrast, has the shortest tendon of the six muscles; for practical purposes it can be thought of as a direct muscular insertion. This muscle inserts lateral to the optic nerve, close to the horizontal meridian, at 9 o'clock for a right eye and 3 o'clock for a left. A critically important structure, the macula, is therefore almost directly interior to the insertion. Surgery involving the inferior oblique muscle must be contemplated with this fact in mind.

Vascular Landmarks

The long posterior ciliary arteries and nerves insert into the sclera close to the optic nerve and proceed anteriorly in the 3 and 9 o'clock meridians. They appear as straight bluish lines on the sclera and are useful for defining the horizontal axis. Normally the nasal artery and nerve are more prominent, because the temporal ones are partially hidden by the inferior oblique muscle (Fig. 3-5).

As any student of anatomy knows, if there are "long" posterior arteries, there must be "short" ones; these form

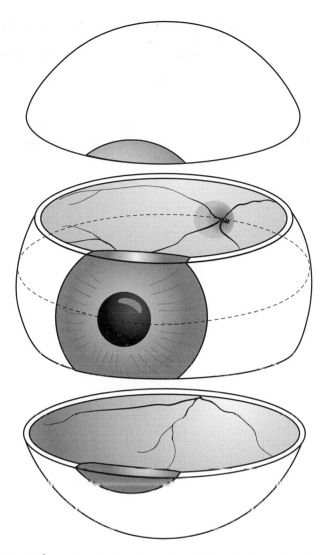

Fig. 3-6 Exploded view of a sectioned eye, showing the central portion, which is submitted for embedding, and the superior and inferior caps, which are not routinely submitted for embedding, but are stored to be retrieved if necessary. The dotted line indicates the ideal microscopic slide section, which includes pupil, optic nerve, and fovea.

MAJOR POINTS

The eye reaches adult size by age 3.

The limbus, a transition between cornea and sclera, is wider in the vertical meridian than the horizontal.

The rectus muscles insert posterior to the limbus and anterior to the equator. Their insertions approximate the anterior extent of the sensory retina.

The oblique muscles insert posterior to the equator. The inferior oblique muscle inserts lateral to the optic nerve and therefore approximately over the macula.

The globe is supplied by the 2 long posterior ciliary arteries, the 10 to 12 short posterior ciliary arteries surrounding the optic nerve, and the 7 anterior ciliary arteries that travel with the rectus muscles.

Sectioning the Eye There are many different proposed methods of sectioning an eye, and which one is used depends in part on the clinical diagnosis and applicable questions. Nonetheless, so-called "routine" sections are taken so that maximal information can be obtained from a single tissue block.

Two parallel cuts are made from back to front, one above and one below the optic nerve, proceeding anteriorly to exit the eye just inside the limbus. In this way, the central portion includes the cornea, anterior chamber, iris and pupil, lens, retina, and optic nerve. If taken horizontally, this central portion will also include the macula (Fig. 3-6). After embedding, this block of tissue is sectioned by microtome to obtain sections through the center of the eye.

If the eye contains a tumor or if there has been previous surgery, it may be preferable to orient these parallel cuts vertically or obliquely. Nonetheless, the central portion still includes all the structures listed above, except the macula.

Alternative methods of sectioning the eye include removing the anterior segment anterior to the ora serrata to show anterior segment structures from behind or to show a clinician's view of the posterior segment. One can also dissect the eye to isolate particular structures; this approach would be particularly applicable for electron microscopic studies or for immunohistochemical or research studies.

SUGGESTED READINGS

Apple DJ, Lim ES, Morgan RC, et al: Preparation and study of human eyes obtained postmortem with the Miyake posterior photographic technique, *Ophthalmology* 97:810-816, 1990.

the vascular annulus of Zinn, entering the sclera around the optic nerve. There are about 10 to 12 of these short posterior ciliary arteries. Moreover, if there are "posterior" arteries, there are also "anterior" ones. There are seven anterior ciliary arteries, each of which travels with a rectus muscle and enters the globe at the attachment of the muscle. All of the rectus muscles have two anterior ciliary arteries, except for the lateral rectus, which only has one.

These anterior ciliary arteries nourish the anterior aspect of the globe. Interference with too many of them, as with overexuberant strabismus surgery, can cause ocular ischemic syndrome.

Custer PL, Trinkaus KM: Volumetric determination of enucleation implant size, *Am J Ophthalmol* 128:489-494, 1999.

Cusumano A, Coleman DJ, Silverman RH, et al: Three-dimensional ultrasound imaging: clinical applications, *Ophthalmology* 105:300-306, 1998.

Ettl A, Kramer J, Daxer A, Koornneef L: High resolution magnetic resonance imaging of neurovascular orbital anatomy, *Ophthalmology* 104:869-877, 1997.

Folberg R, Verdick R, Weingeist TA, Montague PR: The gross examination of eyes removed for choroidal and ciliary body melanomas, *Ophthalmology* 93:1643-1647, 1986.

Hogan MA, Alvarado J, Weddell J: *Histology of the human eye,* Philadelphia, 1971, WB Saunders.

Torczynski E: Preparation of ocular specimens for histopathologic examination, *Ophthalmology* 88:1367-1371, 1981.

White MH, Lambert HM, Kincaid MC, et al: The ora serrata and the spiral of Tillaux: anatomic relationship and clinical correlation, *Ophthalmology* 96:508-511, 1989.

Williamson TH, Harris A: Color Doppler ultrasound imaging of the eye and orbit, *Surv Ophthalmol* 40:255-267, 1996.

Cornea and Sclera: The Outer Coats

CORNEA

How can the cornea, a living tissue, be transparent enough to transmit light? Most living tissue is translucent, but not transparent, certainly not with what we consider to be "optical quality." Several structural and functional adaptations make this ability possible.

Transparency means that there is no significant light scatter. Light rays within the visible spectrum pass through the optical media without being bounced about haphazardly. This lack of scatter of the cornea contrasts with the sclera, for example. Light rays hitting the sclera reflect back in all directions, and no particular visible wavelength is absorbed. Thus sclera therefore appears white.

How does the cornea achieve this quality of transparency? There are several explanations. To begin with, the cornea is avascular. It receives its nutrition by diffusion; the surface is nourished by tears and the inner aspect by the aqueous fluid. There are also no pigmented cells in the cornea. This seems self-evident; yet in some individuals, the conjunctival epithelium is indeed pigmented to some degree, right up to the limbus. These are some of the explanations, but there are additional reasons, anatomic and physiologic, why the cornea is transparent, as explained later in this chapter.

The cornea has a greater radius of curvature than the sclera, and thus it bulges outward. The radius of curvature can be expressed either in millimeters or in diopters of power. The cornea provides two-thirds of the total refractive power of the eye, but unlike the lens, the corneal power is fixed. Centrally, the cornea is just over 0.5 mm thick; it thickens peripherally. The thickness of the cornea in the living eye can be measured optically by corneal pachymetry. Increased thickness can mean increased corneal edema.

Epithelium

The corneal epithelium is physically regular (Fig. 4-1). In contrast to the conjunctival epithelium, with which it is continuous, the basal layer, as well as the surface, is even and parallel to the underlying layers. Thus there is minimal variation in thickness and no undulation of the basal layer. This evenness and regularity help to minimize light scatter.

The epithelium is five to six cell layers in thickness (Fig. 4-2). The cells of the basal layer are low columnar; that is, they are taller than they are wide, so that they are oriented perpendicular to the basal surface. The cells flatten more superficially. The next two to three layers are called wing cells because of their shape. The most superficial two to three layers are flattened surface cells. Like that of the conjunctiva, the corneal epithelium is not keratinized. Numerous microvilli on the surface trap the mucin secreted by the conjunctival goblet cells, allowing the formation of a smooth optical surface.

The epithelium forms a thin basement membrane that overlies Bowman's layer. Like other basement membranes, it is composed of type IV collagen. The epithelial basal layer attaches itself to the basement membrane by forming hemidesmosomes. The normal attachment is quite firm so that it is difficult to remove the epithelium manually. However, in diseases such as diabetes mellitus or map-dot-fingerprint corneal dystrophy, these hemides-

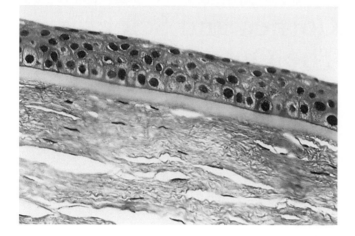

Fig. 4-1   High-power view of corneal epithelium, Bowman's layer, and superficial stroma. There is artifactual separation of stromal lamellae. Hematoxylin and eosin, ×320. (See color plate.)

mosomes are faulty or entirely absent, and thus it is easy to remove the epithelium.

Most surface epithelia lose the superficial layer of cells from chronic exposure and normal wear and tear. New cells are furnished by the basal layer of the epithelium, hence its other name, the germinative layer. However, the corneal epithelium is unusual in that the source of the new cells is not the corneal basal layer, but instead the cells that populate the limbus. These cells are referred to as stem cells. They appear to be responsible for replenishing the corneal epithelial cells and also for preventing the more irregular cells of the adjacent conjunctiva from growing onto the cornea.

Bowman's Layer

The function of Bowman's layer is obscure. It has been theorized that this layer aids in maintaining curvature, yet some animals with corneas having an even greater radius of curvature than the human cornea do not have a Bowman's layer. The origin of this layer is also obscure. It is not a basement membrane, and therefore it is probably preferable to refer to it as a "layer" rather than a "membrane," although both terms are used.

Bowman's layer is acellular (Figs. 4-1 and 4-2). The only cells that normally occupy it are the axons of nerves extending from superficial stroma through it into the epithelium. Peripherally, however, a few fibroblasts may be present. Bowman's layer is composed of type V collagen fibers oriented in random directions, forming a feltwork. This collagen is smaller in diameter (24 to 27 mm) than the collagen of the stroma (32 to 36 mm). Intermixed with the collagen are glycosaminoglycans, forming a

ground substance. By light microscopy Bowman's layer appears uniform and glassy. It is about 8 to 14 μ thick, about 2% of the total corneal thickness.

This layer ends abruptly at the limbus. When it is cut or otherwise damaged, it does not regenerate; instead, the defect is filled by fibrous proliferation or by epithelium.

Stroma

The stroma comprises nearly all of the corneal thickness (Fig. 4-3). The collagen fibers of the stroma are tightly packed and do not branch or terminate within the cornea. These fibers are also highly regular, with a diameter of 32 to 36 mm and a periodicity of 62 to 64 mm. Most of the collagen is type I, with an additional 25% of type VI collagen. Small amounts of types III and V collagen are also present.

The collagen fibers are arranged in discrete lamellae; each layer is oriented differently, so that a given cross section will have layers oriented lengthwise, in cross section, and obliquely. There are about 200 such lamellae, each about 1.5 to 2.5 μ thick.

In between each layer are flattened cells, the keratocytes (Fig. 4-4). They appear inconspicuous by light microscopy. These cells have the characteristics of resting fibrocytes and can be roused to proliferate in the event of injury. In vivo tandem scanning confocal microscopy has shown that there are many more keratocytes than are evident by light microscopy.

In addition to collagen, the stroma contains a number of other proteins and glycoproteins, primarily keratan sulfate, chondroitin, and chondroitin-4-sulfate.

Descemet's Membrane and Endothelium

The endothelium is a remarkable cell layer. It bears the greatest responsibility for maintaining corneal transparency. Although it is called "endothelium" because in certain respects it resembles vascular endothelium, this monolayer of cells arises from the neural crest, rather than from the mesoderm, so it is not truly an endothelium.

At birth, the corneal endothelium has a density of about 3000 cells/mm². It is a monolayer of low cuboidal cells arranged in a hexagonal array and is about 4 to 6 μ thick (Fig. 4-5). However, with time and aging, the endothelium loses cells, because replenishment through mitosis rarely, if ever, occurs. The remaining cells enlarge and become more irregular, a condition known as polymegethism.

The endothelium secretes a thick basement membrane, called Descemet's membrane (Fig. 4-6). By electron microscopy, it is seen to consist of two parts, an

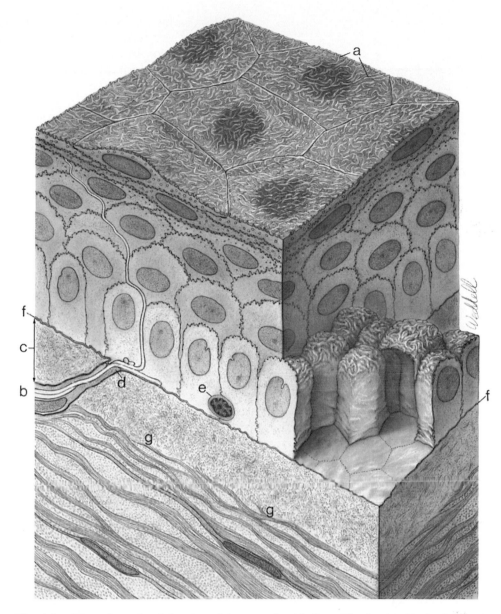

Fig. 4-2   Three-dimensional drawing of the corneal epithelium. The five layers of cells forming this epithelium are shown. The drawing brings out the polygonal shape of the basal and surface cells and their relative size. The wing cell processes fill the spaces formed by the dome-shaped apical surface of the basal cells. The turnover time for these cells is 7 days, and during this time the columnar basal cell is gradually transformed into a wing cell and then into a thin, flat surface cell. During this transition the cytoplasm changes and the Golgi apparatus becomes more prominent. Numerous vesicles develop in the superficial wing and surface layers and glycogen appears in the surface cells. The intercellular space separating the outermost surface cells is closed by a zonula occludens forming a barrier that prevents ingress of the precorneal tear film into the corneal stroma. The cell surface shows an extensive net of microplicae *(a)* and microvilli that may be involved in the retention of the precorneal film. A corneal nerve *(b)* passes through Bowman's layer *(c);* it loses its Schwann sheath near the basement membrane *(d)* of the basal epithelium. The nerve then passes between the epithelial cells toward the superficial layers as a naked nerve. A lymphocyte *(e)* is seen between two basal epithelial cells. The basement membrane is seen at *(f)*. Some of the most superficial corneal stromal lamellae *(g)* are seen curving forward to merge with Bowman's layer. The regular arrangement of the corneal stromal collagen differs from the random disposition of that in Bowman's layer. (From Hogan MA, Alvarado J, Weddell J: *Histology of the human eye*, Philadelphia, 1971, WB Saunders.)

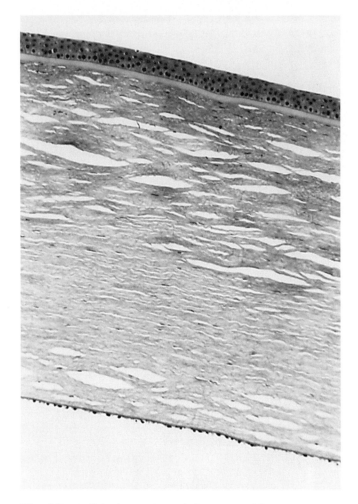

Fig. 4-3 Full-thickness view of the cornea. The stroma comprises the bulk of the total corneal thickness. The stomal lamellae are artifactually separated. Hematoxylin and eosin, ×200 (print magnification).

anterior banded layer, present from birth and unchanging throughout life, and a posterior nonbanded layer, which gradually thickens throughout life. At birth, Descemet's membrane is thinner than the overlying endothelium, whereas in old age it is at least twice as thick.

The endothelium maintains corneal transparency by keeping fluid out of the stroma. The stroma by itself would take up water passively because of the charge characteristics of the mucopolysaccharide matrix. Even with an intact but metabolically inhibited endothelium, some water crosses into the stroma, because the endothelium is a somewhat leaky barrier. How then is the cornea kept at about 70% to 80% water? Contrary to previous speculation, water itself is not actively pumped out. Instead, it follows other ions that are actively pumped out of the cornea into the aqueous. These energy-dependent pumps rely on both aerobic and anaerobic glucose metabolism.

How is this avascular tissue maintained? Toward the periphery, the vascular loops of the limbal capillaries supply nutrition through diffusion. More centrally, the tears are responsible anteriorly and the aqueous posteriorly.

LIMBUS

The limbus forms a transition zone between the transparent cornea and the opaque sclera (Fig. 4-7). Thus it is not a point; it is a region. In this region the collagen diameter increases, and its arrangement becomes less regular.

The posterior boundary of the limbus is a line perpendicular to the sclera going through the angle recess. The anterior boundary joins the termination of Bowman's layer with the termination of Descemet's membrane and the beginning of the trabecular meshwork. By these boundaries, the limbus is about 1.5 mm wide in the horizontal dimension and about 2 mm wide superiorly and inferiorly.

However, histologically it is evident that the boundary between cornea and sclera is not a straight line, but rather is curved, bowed posteriorly at middepth. This line indicates the approximate boundary between the very regular corneal collagen and the more irregular scleral collagen.

SCLERA

The sclera is the tough outer coat of the eye, which gives it support (Fig. 4-8). The scleral thickness varies by region. Adjacent to the limbus, it is just over 0.5 mm in thickness, while at the equator it thins to about 0.4 mm. It is thinner yet behind the rectus muscle insertions. The sclera thickens to 1.0 mm adjacent to the optic nerve. In contrast to that of the cornea, the collagen varies considerably in diameter, from 28 to 280 mm.

The sclera can be divided into three regions, the episclera, the stroma, and the lamina fusca. The episclera is more evident anteriorly. It consists of loose connective tissue along with fibroblasts, elastic tissue, and scattered melanocytes, especially in more pigmented individuals. Vasculature is more prominent in the episclera than in deeper layers. The anterior circulation originates from the anterior ciliary arteries and the posterior circulation from the posterior ciliary vessels.

The scleral stroma consists primarily of type I collagen fibers of varying thickness. Unlike the straight, nonbranching corneal collagen, that of the sclera forms loops and branches. The mucopolysaccharide content of the scleral stroma is low, much lower than that of the

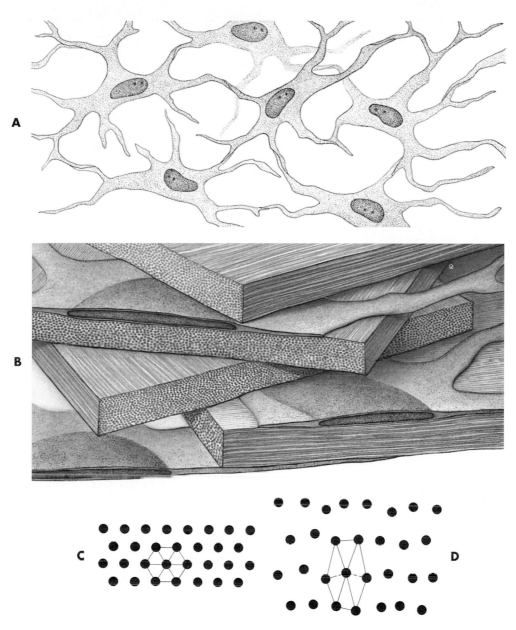

Fig. 4-4   Summary diagram of the corneal stroma. **A,** Fibroblasts. This diagram shows six fibroblasts lying between the stromal lamellae. The cells are thin and flat with long processes which contact fibroblast processes of other cells lying in the same plane. These cells were believed to form a true syncytium, but electron microscopy has disproved this idea. Unlike fibroblasts elsewhere, these cells occasionally join each other at a macula occludens. **B,** Lamellae. The cornea is composed of a very orderly, dense, fibrous connective tissue. Its collagen, which is a very stable protein having a half-life estimated at 100 days, forms many lamellae. The collagen fibrils within a lamella are parallel to each other and run the full length of the cornea. Successive lamellae run across the cornea at an angle to each other. Three fibroblasts are seen between the lamellae. **C,** Diagram to show the theoretical orientation of the corneal collagen fibrils. Each of the fibrils is separated from its fellows by an equal distance. Maurice has explained the transparency of the cornea on the basis of this very exact equidistant separation. As a result of this arrangement the stromal lamellae form a three-dimensional array of diffraction gratings. Scattered rays of light passing through such a system interact with each other in an organized way, resulting in the elimination of scattered light by destructive interference. The mucoproteins, glycoproteins and other components of the ground substance are responsible for maintaining the proper position of the fibrils. **D,** Orientation of the collagen fibrils in an opaque cornea. The diagram shows the orderly positions of the fibrils to have been disturbed. Because of this disarrangement, scattered light is not eliminated by destructive interference and the cornea becomes hazy. (From Hogan MA, Alvarado J, Weddell J: *Histology of the human eye,* Philadelphia, 1971, WB Saunders.)

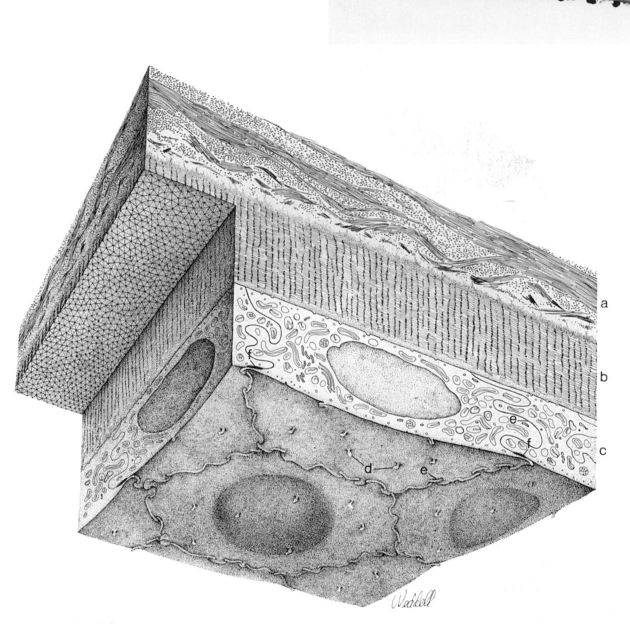

Fig. 4-5 High-power view of Descemet's membrane and endothelium. In this young patient, the endothelium is slightly thicker than Descemet's membrane. Hematoxylin and eosin, ×320. (See color plate.)

Fig. 4-6 Three-dimensional drawing of the deep cornea showing the deepest corneal lamellae *(a)*, Descemet's membrane *(b)*, and the endothelium *(c)*. The deeper stromal lamellae split, and some branches curve posteriorly to merge with Descemet's membrane. Descemet's membrane is seen in meridional and tangential planes. The endothelial cells are polygonal in shape, measuring approximately 3.5 mm in thickness and 7 to 10 mm in length. Microvilli *(d)* protrude into the anterior chamber from the posterior cell, and the marginal folds *(e)* at intercellular junctions project into the anterior chamber. The intercellular space near the anterior chamber is closed by a zonula occludens *(f)*. The cytoplasm contains an abundance of rod-shaped mitochondria. The nucleus is round and flattened in the anteroposterior axis. (From Hogan MA, Alvarado J, Weddell J: *Histology of the human eye,* Philadelphia, 1971, WB Saunders.)

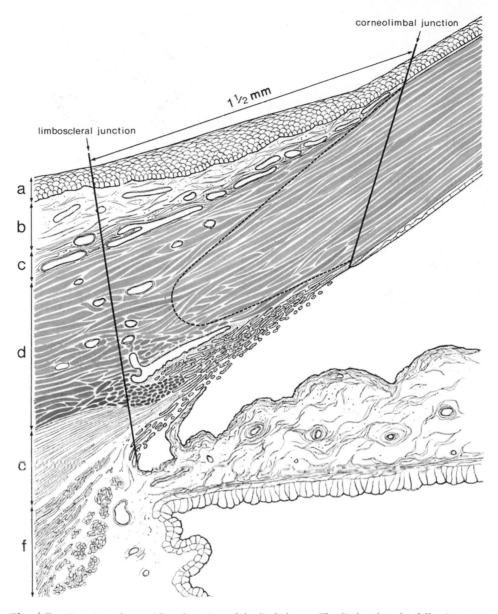

Fig. 4-7   Drawing of a meridional section of the limbal area. The limbus has the following gross anatomic parts: Conjunctival epithelium *(a)*, conjunctival stroma *(b)*, Tenon's capsule and episclera *(c)*, and the limbal or corneoscleral stroma *(d)*. The longitudinal portion of the ciliary muscle is indicated at *e* and circular and radial bundles of the muscle at *f*. The microscopic subdivisions of the limbus are seen in Fig. 4-9. (From Hogan MA, Alvarado J, Weddell J: *Histology of the human eye,* Philadelphia, 1971, WB Saunders.)

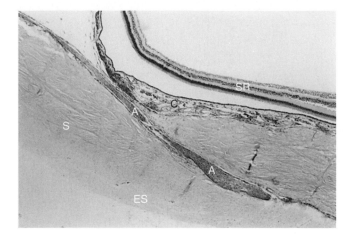

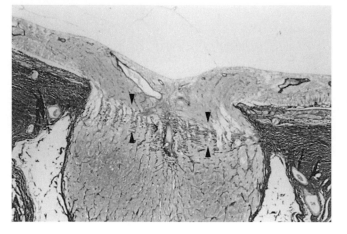

Fig. 4-8   One of the long posterior ciliary arteries *(A)* enters the sclera *(S)* and traverses its entire thickness to enter beneath the choroid *(C)*. The overlying retina *(SR)* is artifactually detached. The episclera *(ES)* does not have an abrupt boundary, but appears paler and less dense on staining. Hematoxylin and eosin, ×20. (See color plate.)

Fig. 4-9   The sclera is continuous with the lamina cribrosa *(arrowheads)* through which the optic nerve exits the eye. Gomori methenamine silver, ×20. (See color plate.)

cornea. Also present are small amounts of elastic tissue. The stroma is relatively acellular and avascular, but there are vascular channels, most notably for the long posterior ciliary arteries at the horizontal meridians, the short posterior ciliary arteries, and the vortex veins. Especially in more darkly pigmented individuals, these channels may be lined by melanocytes.

The lamina fusca is a thin layer of collagen fibers and melanocytes that serves to anchor the choroid and ciliary body to the sclera.

The sclera becomes continuous with the dura surrounding the optic nerve. However, it also changes to form a sieve-like opening for the exit of the optic nerve (Fig. 4-9). This structure is the lamina cribrosa, which consists of several connective tissue plates with perforations.

MAJOR POINTS

The cornea's transparency is explained by its orderly structure, its avascularity, and the pumping action of the endothelium that keeps it relatively dehydrated.

The cornea receives nutrition from the vascular arcades at the limbus, the tears anteriorly, and the aqueous posteriorly.

The corneal epithelium is orderly and regular. Unlike other epithelia, its cells are replenished not by the basal layer of the corneal epithelium, but by the stem cells of the limbus.

Bowman's layer is of uncertain origin and function. It is an acellular, glassy layer composed of a feltwork of collagen fibers. It does not regenerate after damage, but instead any defect is filled by epithelial cells or fibrous proliferation.

The corneal stroma centrally is just over 0.5 mm thick and is composed of collagen and mucopolysaccharides. The collagen fibers are regular in diameter and do not branch or terminate within the stroma. They are arranged in lamellae of different orientations.

The keratocytes are a type of resting fibrocytes between the collagen lamellae of the stroma.

The corneal endothelium secretes Descemet's membrane, a thick basement membrane that consists of two parts. The posterior part gradually thickens throughout life.

The corneal endothelium originates from the neural crest. Via several energy-requiring enzyme systems, it pumps ions out of the cornea into the aqueous. Water follows these ions passively.

At the limbus, the transition zone between cornea and sclera, the collagen becomes more irregular in diameter and arrangement. It is about 2 mm wide superiorly and inferiorly and about 1.5 mm wide laterally and medially.

The sclera supports the ocular contents, imparting a certain degree of rigidity. It is thickest around the optic nerve, where it becomes continuous with the dura, and thinnest just behind the rectus insertions. The stromal collagen is much less regular in arrangement and thickness than that of the cornea, accounting for its opacity.

The sclera is modified to form the lamina cribrosa posteriorly, through which the axons of the optic nerve exit the eye.

SUGGESTED READINGS

Bahn CF, Sugar A: Endothelial physiology and intraocular lens implantation, *Am Intra-Ocular Implant Soc J* 7:351-364, 1981.

Daxer A, Misof K, Grabner B, et al: Collagen fibrils in the human corneal stroma: structure and aging, *Invest Ophthalmol Vis Sci* 39:644-648, 1998.

Doughty MJ, Zaman ML: Human corneal thickness and its impact on intraocular pressure measures: a review and meta-analysis approach, *Surv Ophthalmol* 44:367-408, 2000.

Dua HS, Azuara-Blanco A: Limbal stem cells of the corneal epithelium, *Surv Ophthalmol* 44:415-425, 2000.

Hirst LW, Green WR, Kues HA: Clinical specular microscopic/pathologic correlation, *Cornea* 2:159-164,1983.

Murphy C, Alvarado J, Juster R, Maglio M: Prenatal and postnatal cellularity of the human corneal endothelium, *Invest Ophthalmol Vis Sci* 25:312-322, 1984.

Murphy C, Alvarado J, Juster R: Prenatal and postnatal growth of the human Descemet's membrane, *Invest Ophthalmol Vis Sci* 25:1402-1415, 1984.

Olsen TW, Aaberg SY, Geroski DH, Edelhauser HF: Human sclera: thickness and surface area, *Am J Ophthalmol* 125: 237-241, 1998.

Shamsuddin AKM, Nirankari VS, Purnell DM, Chang SH: Is the corneal posterior cell layer truly endothelial? *Ophthalmology* 93:1298-1303, 1986.

Waring GW III, Bourne WM, Edelhauser HF, Kenyon KR: The corneal endothelium: normal and pathologic structure and function, *Ophthalmology* 89:53 1-590, 1982.

Williams KK, Noe RL, Grossniklaus HE, et al: Correlation of histologic corneal endothelial cell counts with specular microscopic cell density, *Arch Ophthalmol* 110:1146-1149, 1992.

Tears: The Ins and Outs

Most surface epithelium of the body is keratinized as a protective device. Yet for the eye, keratinization is clearly not suitable. The ocular surface is covered with mucosa and is therefore kept constantly moist. However, moisturization is more difficult for the eye than for other mucosal surfaces. Unlike a typical mucosa, which is protected from the air, the eye must be exposed to function. Maintaining clarity and moisture is the function of the eyelids and the tears. Protection of the eye, along with clearance of the tears, is the function of the eyelids.

TEAR LAYERS

We tend to think of tears as simply salty water. However, tears are actually quite complex, and their composition depends on the interaction of several secretory glands (Fig. 5-1).

Tears have several functions. They must create a smooth optical surface for optimal vision. Also they hydrate the nonkeratinized ocular surface and supply oxygen and nutrients to the corneal epithelium. In ad-

dition, the tears act as a barrier to infection, since they contain considerable quantities of immunoglobulins, primarily IgA.

Mucin Layer

Tears are largely water, yet the unit membrane of a cell, including the surface cell layer of the cornea and conjunctiva, is hydrophobic because it is composed of lipid subunits. Therefore there must be a wetting agent to allow the tears to adhere properly. This wetting agent is mucin, a mucopolysaccharide, secreted by the goblet cells of the conjunctiva. This mucin binds to the microvilli of the corneal and conjunctival surface and can be seen by electron microscopy as a fuzzy substance called the glycocalyx, about 0.5 μ thick. Abnormal or deficient mucin prevents the tear film from spreading over the cornea properly.

Goblet cells (Fig. 5-2) are single cell glands residing in the conjunctival epithelium. Histologically they are oval to round in shape and are paler than the surrounding epithelium. The goblet cell population varies by location; they are most numerous in the fornices and their number also increases considerably as one goes from temporal to nasal.

Aqueous Layer

The thickest layer of the tears is the aqueous layer, approximately 6 to 8 μ in thickness. The aqueous component of tears is secreted by the main lacrimal gland and the accessory glands in the eyelid, the glands of Wolfring and Krause.

The main lacrimal gland lies in the anterior orbit, superotemporal to the globe. It is divided into two parts, the palpebral lobe, located laterally in the upper lid, and the orbital lobe. The duct from the orbital portion proceeds inferiorly through the palpebral lobe.

Both the main and the accessory glands are similar in structure, classified as compound acinar glands (Fig. 5-3). Individual acini have two cell layers, an outer flattened myoepithelial layer and an inner secretory layer. The latter consists of cuboidal cells surrounding a central lumen. Several acini empty their contents into small ducts, which join ultimately to form the main duct.

The accessory lacrimal glands are located in the fornices and at the tarsal margins. The forniceal glands are also called the glands of Krause, and number about 40 in the upper lid, but only 6 to 8 in the lower. There are fewer glands of Wolfring on the tarsal margins; they number up to 5 in the upper lid and 2 in the lower. Unlike the main lacrimal gland, which receives parasympathetic innervation, they are not innervated. Some authorities postulate that these accessory glands therefore supply the basal tear secretion, whereas the main lacrimal gland supplies reflex secretion.

The tears contain a considerable amount of protein, including a modified albumin that acts as a buffer, interferon, and immunoglobulin A. The levels of most of the small molecules and ions, such as urea and amino acids, are similar to those in blood plasma. However, there is less glucose and more potassium and chloride.

Lipid Layer

The outermost layer is a thin lipid layer, approximately 0.5 μ. A number of lipids, including cholesterol esters, phospholipids, waxes, and triglycerides, make up this layer. It adds stability to the tear film and also appears to inhibit evaporation. The Meibomian glands of the tarsus secrete this layer, with contributions from the Zeis glands, the sebaceous glands of the cilia.

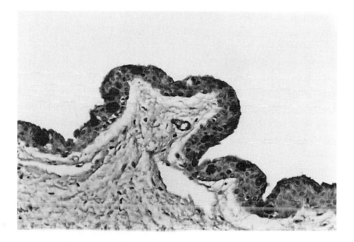

Fig. 5-2 Conjunctiva, near the fornix, showing numerous darkly staining goblet cells in the epithelium. Periodic acid-Schiff, ×200. (See color plate.)

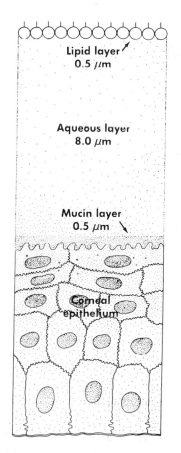

Fig. 5-1 Schema of the precorneal tear film. The mucin is a wetting agent that wets the corneal epithelium. (From Newell FW: *Ophthalmology: principles and concepts,* ed 7, St Louis, 1992, Mosby.)

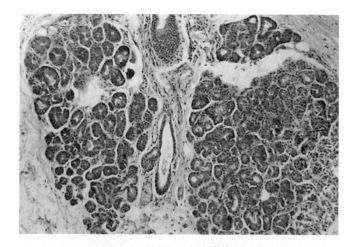

Fig. 5-3 Lacrimal gland, with numerous acini and a central duct. Periodic acid-Schiff, ×78.

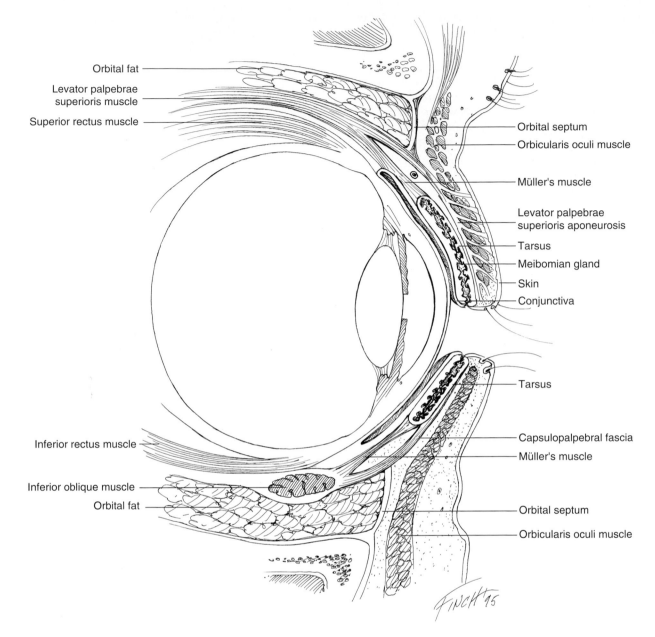

Fig. 5-4   Sagittal section of the upper and lower eyelid. (From Krachmer J, editor: *Cornea*, vol 1, St Louis, 1997, Mosby.)

EYELID

Skin and Subcutaneous Tissue

The eyelid appears to be simply a flap of skin with lashes. Yet, it is exquisitely constructed to allow it to fulfill specific functions (Fig. 5-4). One of these functions is to regulate the amount of light entering the eye. Another is to spread the tear film over the surface of the eye. To prevent evaporation of the tears, the lids blink about 20 times a minute, so rapidly that normally we are unaware of the process. Blinking is also a protective reaction; the lids reflexly close to avoid threatening movements.

The surface of the lid is thin skin, covered with very fine lanugo hairs. The epithelium is keratinized stratified squamous, with the typical layers seen in skin elsewhere. The basal epithelial cell layer is also called the germinative layer; the more superficial cells originate from it. The basal cells are taller than they are wide, with relatively scant cytoplasm. Superficial to the basal layer is the prickle cell layer. Here, the epithelial cells form numerous tight junctions with each other. These are technically known as maculae adherentes, or gap junctions, and can

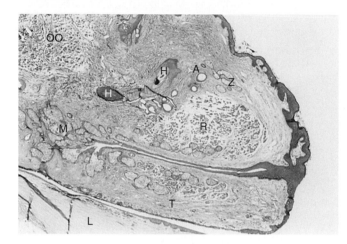

Fig. 5-5   The eyelid. The orbicularis oculi *(OO)* is seen at the upper left. Hair follicles of the lashes *(H)*, with nearby apocrine glands of Moll *(A)* and sebaceous glands of Zeis *(Z)* are seen. Below these is the muscle of Riolan *(R)*. Below this is the tarsus *(T)* which contains a Meibomian gland *(M)* with a prominent duct. Peripheral cornea and limbus *(L)* are seen below. Hematoxylin and eosin, ×20. (See color plate.)

be thought of as "spot welds" binding one cell to the next. By light microscopy, after formalin fixation, these junctions can be seen as innumerable thin lines perpendicular to each cell's surface. Formalin fixation of the tissue causes a slight shrinkage of the cells. Thus the junctions are put on stretch, causing the appearance of these lines. Similar junctions are seen in the corneal and conjunctival epithelium.

Superficial to the prickle cell layer is the granular cell layer. The cells of this layer are considerably flattened. The granules are large, irregular basophilic granules in the cytoplasm and are the precursors to keratin. The keratin layer consists of cells that have lost their nuclei.

There is only a minimal subcutaneous tissue in the lids, within which are the adnexal structures, including fine hairs, sebaceous glands, and eccrine sweat glands.

Cilia

At the lid margin, the cilia or eyelashes are the most striking feature (Fig. 5-5). These act as sensors, triggering a protective blink reflex when touched. The cilia form two to three rows, with more in the upper lid than the lower. As with all hairs, there are associated sebaceous glands. These are the glands of Zeis, surrounding each hair follicle.

Sebaceous glands are present throughout the body, and form part of the hair shaft apparatus. These are holocrine glands, which means that the entire cell becomes the secretory product. Thus the glands have the overall structure of acinar glands, but with no lumen in the cen-

ter of the acinus. Rather, the cells move centrally from the basal, or germinative, layer and become very large, with abundant pale, lipid-laden cytoplasm. The secretory product, sebum, lubricates the hair shaft.

Also in the vicinity are sweat glands, the glands of Moll. These are apocrine sweat glands. They are considerably larger than eccrine sweat glands; however, their general structure, a simple coiled tube, is similar. Both eccrine and apocrine glands have a double epithelium. The outer layer is a flattened myoepithelium, whereas the inner layer is a cuboidal epithelium that secretes the sweat. Apocrine glands pinch off the apex of the cell into the lumen along with the fluid sweat.

Orbicularis Oculi

Deep to the subcutaneous tissue is the orbicularis oculi muscle. This is a striated muscle arranged in an ellipse, whose function is to close the lid. In so doing, it also pulls the puncta and expands the lacrimal sac, forcing tears from the lacrimal lake into the canaliculi. A portion of the orbicularis is separate and lies near the lid margin on both sides of the tarsus; this portion is the muscle of Riolan. The orbicularis oculi is innervated by cranial nerve VII.

Tarsus

On the lid margin, anterior to the Meibomian orifices, is the gray line. This is a cleavage plane; incisions here split the lid between the orbicularis oculi and the tarsus, or tarsal plate. The tarsus is a semicircular structure superiorly, and a narrower, more nearly rectangular structure inferiorly (Fig. 5-6). Each tarsus connects to the medial and lateral canthal tendons, which anchor the lids to the orbit.

The tarsus consists of dense fibrous connective tissue and elastic tissue, within which are the Meibomian glands. There are about 25 of these specialized sebaceous glands in the upper tarsus and 20 in the lower tarsus.

The Meibomian gland is unique in that normally it has no associated hair shaft, and the chemical composition of its sebum is somewhat different from that of ordinary sebaceous glands. We can see these glands clinically at the slit lamp upon eversion of the lids. They appear as yellowish, slightly irregular vertical columns in the tarsus. The gland orifices are visible on the posterior aspect of the lid margin.

Conjunctiva

The conjunctiva is a stratified columnar epithelium, which is loose and redundant in the fornices (Fig. 5-7), but which is tightly apposed to the tarsus. The palpebral

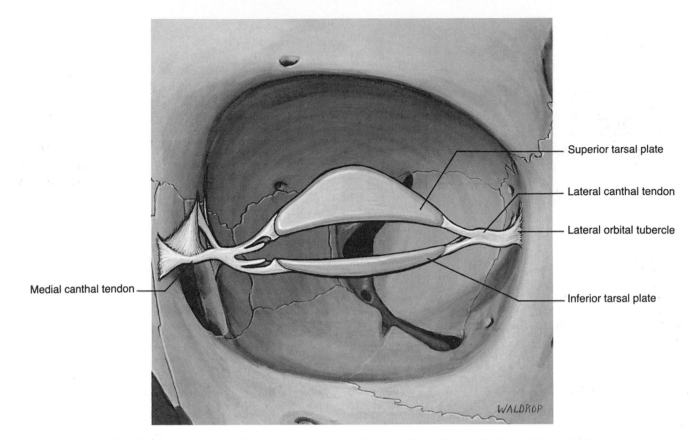

Fig. 5-6   Eyelids, deep dissection of structural elements. (From Dutton JJ: *Atlas of clinical and surgical orbital anatomy,* Philadelphia, 1994, WB Saunders.) (See color plate.)

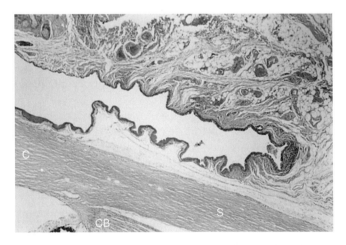

Fig. 5-7   The fornix. The conjunctiva is loose and redundant here, and becomes more adherent at the limbus. The cornea *(C)* is seen to the left, and the sclera *(S)* to the right. A portion of ciliary body *(CB)* is also present. Hematoxylin and eosin, ×20. (See color plate.)

conjunctiva is continuous with the skin at the lid margin. It reflects back at the fornix to form the bulbar conjunctiva, in turn becoming continuous with the corneal epithelium. The superior fornix is considerably deeper than the inferior fornix. Adjacent to the limbus and to the eyelid margin, the conjunctiva becomes stratified squamous, as a transition to corneal epithelium and lid skin, respectively.

Subjacent to the epithelium is the loose connective tissue stroma, which is richly vascularized. Lymphatics are also present; those anterior to the tarsus drain to the preauricular nodes and those posterior drain to the submandibular nodes. There is also a resident population of lymphocytes. At the limbus and over the tarsus, however, the stroma is compact and very thin. Firm connections anchor the conjunctiva at these locations.

The blood supply to the conjunctiva comes from branches of both the ophthalmic and facial arteries. At the limbus, terminal vessels loop toward the cornea, forming the palisades of Vogt.

The caruncle is a specialized structure that lies at the nasal extreme of the conjunctiva. The epithelium is similar to that of the conjunctiva, but the stroma is denser. Several hair follicles with fine hairs and sebaceous glands occupy the stroma, sometimes along with an accessory lacrimal gland. Just lateral to the caruncle is the semilunar fold, analogous to the nictitating membrane in lower animals. In the human, it appears to function simply as another redundant fold in the conjunctiva, allowing free movement of the eyeball.

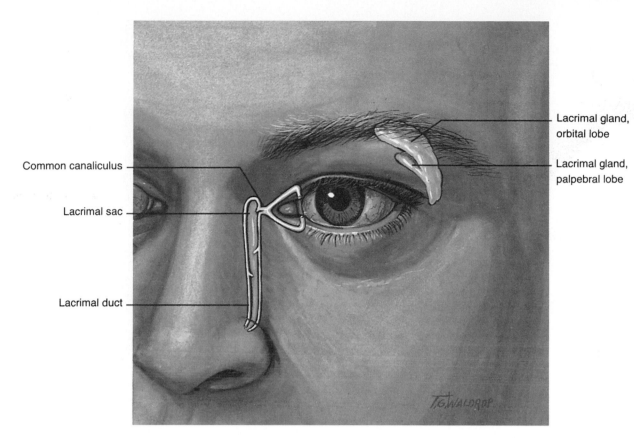

Common canaliculus

Lacrimal sac

Lacrimal duct

Lacrimal gland, orbital lobe

Lacrimal gland, palpebral lobe

Fig. 5-8   Lacrimal systems. (From Dutton JJ: *Atlas of clinical and surgical orbital anatomy,* Philadelphia, 1994, WB Saunders.) (See color plate.)

Eyelid Musculature

The levator muscle raises the upper lid. It originates at the orbital apex and comes anteriorly along with, and above, the superior rectus muscle. Like the superior rectus, it is innervated by cranial nerve III. Its aponeurosis descends to insert into the upper lid, anterior to the tarsus, with numerous fibrous strands coming through the orbicularis muscle to insert into the subcutaneous tissue. The levator aponeurosis also fuses to the orbital septum.

Müller's muscle lies posterior to the aponeurosis of the levator muscle and inserts into the superior tarsal margin. Müller's muscle is smooth muscle, innervated by the sympathetic system. Thus when the sympathetic system is generally stimulated, as when a person is surprised or angry, the upper eyelid elevates 1 to 2 mm. Laterally, Müller's muscle splits and passes and surrounds the palpebral lobe of the lacrimal gland. Müller's muscle of the lower lid inserts into the inferior margin of the lower tarsus and has an action similar to that of the upper lid.

The orbital septum is a thin fibrous membrane at the level of the orbital rim. Structures posterior to it are considered intraorbital.

LACRIMAL DRAINAGE

Because tears are constantly produced, they must also be constantly drained. They exit from the ocular surface via the canaliculi and ultimately enter the nose beneath the inferior turbinate.

Canaliculi

On the medial aspect of each eyelid is a small hole, the punctum. It is apposed to the globe, but can easily be reflected back for examination. This is the opening for the canaliculus, and it is surrounded by a ring of connective tissue and striated muscle fibers.

Each canaliculus is about 0.5 mm in diameter (Fig. 5-8). It is oriented approximately vertically for a short distance, then it proceeds medially and posteriorly about 8 mm. The upper and lower canaliculi meet to form the common canaliculus, which drains into the lacrimal sac. The canaliculi are lined by a nonkeratinized stratified squamous epithelium. Like the puncta, the canaliculi are surrounded by connective tissue and muscle fibers from the muscle of Riolan of the orbicularis oculi muscle (Fig. 5-9).

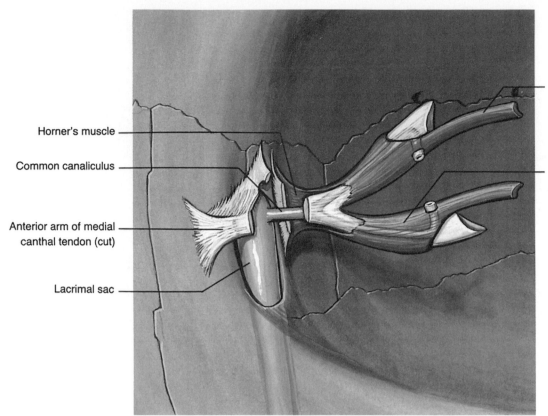

Horner's muscle

Common canaliculus

Anterior arm of medial
canthal tendon (cut)

Lacrimal sac

Superior muscle of
Riolan

Deep head of inferior
pretarsal orbicularis
muscle

Fig. 5-9   Lacrimal drainage system, superficial anatomy. (From Dutton JJ: *Atlas of clinical and surgical orbital anatomy,* Philadelphia, 1994, WB Saunders.) (See color plate.)

Tears are forced into the canaliculi by the blinking action of the lids, which sweep the tears medially. The orbicularis muscle fibers keep the puncta open, and the suction effect created draws the tears in.

Lacrimal Sac

The lacrimal sac lies in the lacrimal fossa, medial to the globe. The fossa is formed by the lacrimal bone and a portion of the maxilla. The periorbital connective tissue surrounds the sac. It is lined by stratified columnar epithelium with goblet cells, and sometimes also with cilia, like respiratory epithelium.

Lacrimal Duct

The sac empties into the lacrimal duct, which is somewhat narrower and which has folds in the mucosa. The duct is about 12 mm long and descends within a bony canal to empty into the nose beneath the inferior turbinate. The mucosal folds, collectively called Hasner's valve, minimize retrograde flow of mucus or air.

SUGGESTED READINGS

Doane MG: Blinking and the mechanics of the lacrimal drainage system, *Ophthalmology* 88:844-851, 1981.

Farris RL, Stuchell RN, Mandel ID: Basal and reflex human tear analysis. I. Physical measurements: osmolarity, basal volumes, and reflex flow rate, *Ophthalmology* 88:852-857, 1981.

Goldberg RA, Wu JC, Jesmanowicz A, Hyde JS: Eyelid anatomy revisited: dynamic high-resolution magnetic resonance images of Whitnall's ligament and upper eyelid structures with the use of a surface coil, *Arch Ophthalmology* 110:1598-1600, 1992.

Jeong S, Lemke BN, Dortzvach RK, et al: The Asian upper eyelid: an anatomical study with comparison to the Caucasian eyelid, *Arch Ophthalmol* 117:907-912, 1999.

Kinoshita S, Kiorpes TC, Friend J, Thoft RA: Goblet cell density in ocular surface disease: a better indicator than tear mucin, *Arch Ophthalmol* 101:1284-1287, 1983.

Maskin SL, Bodé DD: Electron microscopy of impression-acquired conjunctival epithelial cells, *Ophthalmology* 93: 1518-1523, 1986.

Obata H, Yamamoto S, Horiuchi H, Machinami R: Histopathologic study of human lacrimal gland: statistical analysis with

MAJOR POINTS

The tears consist of three layers, the innermost mucin layer secreted by the conjunctival goblet cells, the aqueous layer secreted by the main and accessory lacrimal glands, and the lipid layer, secreted by the Meibomian glands.

The mucin modifies the cell surface of the cornea, which would otherwise be hydrophobic, allowing uniform wetting.

Immunoglobulin A and interferon are secreted in the aqueous portion of the tears; they help prevent infection.

The accessory lacrimal glands, located at the tarsal margins and the fornices, are not innervated, while the lacrimal gland receives parasympathetic innervation. Histologically, all the glands are compound acinar glands.

The Meibomian glands are sebaceous glands located within the tarsus of both upper and lower lids. Unlike other sebaceous glands, no hair shafts are normally associated with them.

Sebaceous glands are holocrine glands. The entire cell material of the acinus is discharged into the duct.

The conjunctival epithelium is continuous with both the corneal epithelium and the skin of the lid. Except at the limbus and over the tarsus, it is loose and redundant, allowing free movement of the globe. Goblet cells, single-cell glands, are most numerous in the fornices and nasally.

Lymphocytes normally reside in the conjunctival stroma, where they may form follicles.

The levator muscle, innervated by cranial nerve III, raises the upper lid, while the orbicularis, innervated by cranial nerve VII, closes the lids. Both lids have a Müller's muscle, innervated by the sympathetic system, that widens the interpalpebral fissure.

Tears exit the ocular surface through the puncta. The lids sweep the tears medially, and the orbicularis muscle fibers open the puncta, creating a suction effect. The tears enter the nasopharynx beneath the inferior turbinate.

special reference to aging, *Ophthalmology* 102:678-686, 1995.

Stuchell RN, Farris RL, Mandel ID: Basal and reflex human tear analysis. II. Chemical analysis: lactoferrin and lysozyme, *Ophthalmology* 88:858-862, 1988.

Tucker NA, Tucker SM, Linberg JV: The anatomy of the common canaliculus, *Arch Ophthalmol* 114:1231-1234, 1996.

Watanabe H, Maeda N, Kiritoshi A, et al: Expression of a mucin-like glycoprotein produced by ocular surface epithelium in normal and keratinized cells, *Am J Ophthalmol* 124:751-757, 1997.

Wieczorek R, Jakobiec RA, Sacks EH, Knowles DM: The immunoarchitecture of the normal human lacrimal gland. relevancy for understanding pathologic conditions, *Ophthalmology* 95:100-109, 1988.

Wright P: Normal tear production and drainage, *Trans Ophthalmol Soc UK* 104:351-354, 1985.

CHAPTER 6

Aqueous: The Inner Circulation

The transparent cornea and lens are both living structures but are avascular. How do they obtain nutrition and discard metabolic waste? For the ocular media to refract light, not only must the living tissue remain transparent, so must the ocular fluids that bathe the ocular structures. The aqueous, the constantly circulating fluid responsible for nourishing the inner aspect of cornea, trabecular meshwork, and the anterior portion of the lens, must therefore convey oxygen and nutrients and carry away metabolic waste products, all without benefit of red cells or even protein.

Moreover, the aqueous fluid and the resistance to its outflow are responsible for maintaining the intraocular pressure of the eye. In turn, this intraocular pressure itself helps maintain the transparency of the ocular tissues. If intraocular pressure in an eye is too low corneal haze and refractive instability develop.

FORMATION AND DRAINAGE OF THE AQUEOUS

The aqueous fluid is a watery fluid that normally is acellular. It is analogous to the cerebrospinal fluid that surrounds the central nervous system, although it is not chemically identical with it. Compared with serum, the aqueous contains about two-thirds the amount of glucose, far less protein, but much more ascorbate and lactate.

Ciliary Epithelium

The aqueous is derived from blood plasma, which crosses the capillary walls into the parenchyma of the ciliary processes by ultrafiltration (Fig. 6-1). The capillaries of the ciliary processes are large, dilated vessels, 20 to 30 μ in diameter, with large pores. The plasma solutes are taken up selectively from the parenchyma into the ciliary body pigmented epithelium and then are transferred across into the nonpigmented epithelium where they are actively secreted by the cells as aqueous fluid. The take up and secretion across the cell membranes occur via active transport. Water passively follows the ions and other materials that are actively secreted.

Several substances decrease aqueous fluid secretion, including β-blockers, prostaglandins, epinephrine and its analogs, and carbonic anhydrase inhibitors.

Intraocular Circulation

Once it crosses the basement membrane of the non-pigmented epithelium, the aqueous enters the posterior chamber at a rate of 2 to 3 μL/min. The posterior chamber is bounded by the lens capsule and anterior zonules posteriorly, the posterior surface of the iris anteriorly, and the ciliary processes laterally.

After entering the posterior chamber, the aqueous goes between iris and lens to enter the anterior chamber via the pupil. It then exits the eye at the trabecular meshwork.

The anterior chamber is considerably larger than the posterior chamber. It is bounded by the cornea anteriorly, the trabecular meshwork laterally, and the anterior surfaces of the iris and lens posteriorly. At its deepest, centrally, the anterior chamber is about 3.5 mm deep, but this depth varies from person to person and also

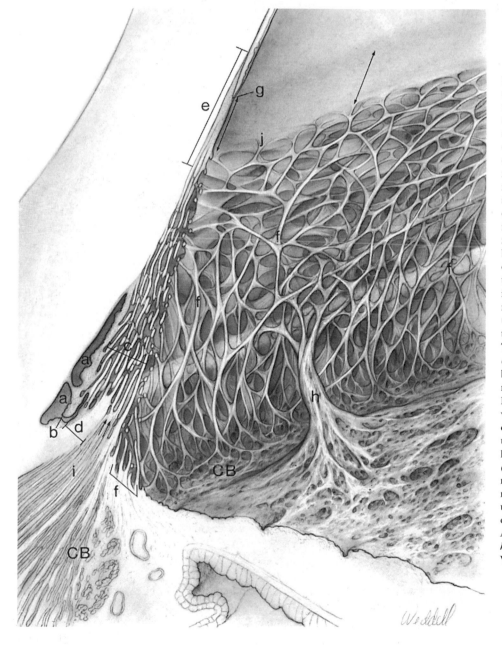

Fig. 6-1   Low-power view of the anterior segment. The lens *(L)* is at the lower left. To the right are the processes of the ciliary body *(CB)*. These two structures, along with the posterior surface of the iris *(I)*, define the posterior chamber. Anteriorly is the cornea *(C)*. Schlemm's canal *(S)* is readily seen, just to the right of the trabecular meshwork. Hematoxylin and eosin, ×20. (See color plate.)

Fig. 6-2   Drawing of the aqueous outflow apparatus and adjacent tissues. Schlemm's canal *(a)* is divided into two portions. An internal collector channel (Sondermann) *(b)* opens into the posterior part of the canal. The sheets of the corneoscleral meshwork *(c)* extend from the corneolimbus *(e)* anteriorly to the scleral spur *(d)*. The ropelike components of the uveal meshwork *(f)* occupy the inner portion of the trabecular meshwork; they arise in the ciliary body *(CB)* near the angle recess and end just posterior to the termination of Descemet's membrane *(g)*. An iris process *(h)* extends from the root of the iris to merge with the uveal meshwork at about the level of the anterior part of the scleral spur. The longitudinal ciliary muscle *(i)* is attached to the scleral spur but has a portion that joins the corneoscleral meshwork *(arrows)*. Descemet's membrane terminates within the deep corneolimbus. The corneal endothelium becomes continuous with the trabecular endothelium *(j)*. A broad transition zone *(double-headed arrows)* begins near the termination of Descemet's membrane and ends where the uveal meshwork joins the deep corneolimbus. (From Hogan MA, Alvarado J, Weddell J: *Histology of the human eye,* Philadelphia, 1971, WB Saunders.)

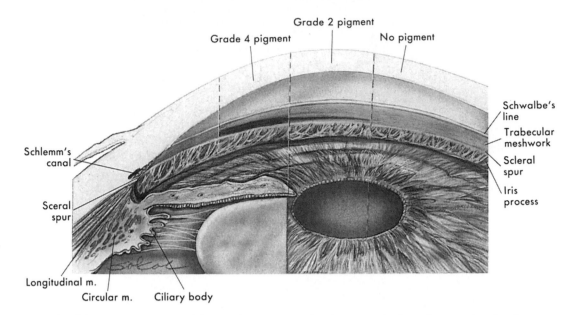

Fig. 6-3   Schematic view of the zonules separating the vitreous cavity from the posterior chamber and the iris separating the anterior and posterior chambers. (From Hoskins HD, Kass M: *Becker-Shaffer's diagnosis and treatment of the glaucomas,* ed 6, St Louis, 1989, Mosby.)

decreases with age, as the lens grows. Normally, the iris is planar from pupil to iris root.

Trabecular Meshwork

The trabecular meshwork is a roughly triangular structure bounded by the periphery of the cornea anteriorly and by the scleral spur and anterior surface of the ciliary body posteriorly (Fig. 6-2). It is a sieve of connective tissue and elastic tissue strands covered by endothelial cells, which are continuous with corneal endothelium.

The termination of Descemet's membrane is called Schwalbe's line, and there is often a variable amount of fibrous tissue proliferation here. Clinically, by gonioscopy, Schwalbe's line is a thin, bright line at the peripheral margin of the cornea (Fig. 6-3). The anterior margin of the trabecular meshwork inserts here. The trabecular meshwork consists of two parts, the corneoscleral mesh and the uveoscleral mesh. Clinically, the meshwork is pale tan to dark brown, depending on the amount of pigmentation.

The corneoscleral mesh is the more external (Fig. 6-4). The meshwork is more solid here, with smaller pores and a more sheetlike parenchyma. The openings are about 12 to 20 μ in diameter and are not in register; thus exit through the meshwork is tortuous. Anteriorly, at Schwalbe's line, there are only 2 to 3 layers, which increase to about 10 to 12 layers going posteriorly. The posterior margin of the corneoscleral trabecular meshwork is bounded by the scleral spur. This is a variably prominent inward extension of sclera to which the longitudinal muscle of the ciliary body attaches on the pos-

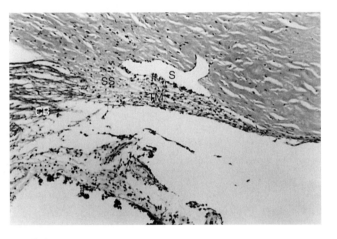

Fig. 6-4   The corneoscleral meshwork *(TM)* and Schlemm's canal *(S).* The longitudinal muscle of the ciliary body *(CB)* inserts into scleral spur *(SS).* The uveoscleral mesh and the iris are artifactually disrupted. Trichrome, ×80. (See color plate.)

terior side. Clinically, it is a broad, bright band at the posterior margin of the trabecular meshwork.

The most inward portion of the trabecular meshwork bypasses the scleral spur and inserts directly onto the anterior face of the ciliary body. This is the uveoscleral meshwork, and the individual beams are more ropelike, creating larger pores. This portion consists of only about 2 to 3 layers.

Schlemm's Canal

Schlemm's canal is the drainage site where much of the aqueous exits the eye (Fig. 6-5). It is an elongated

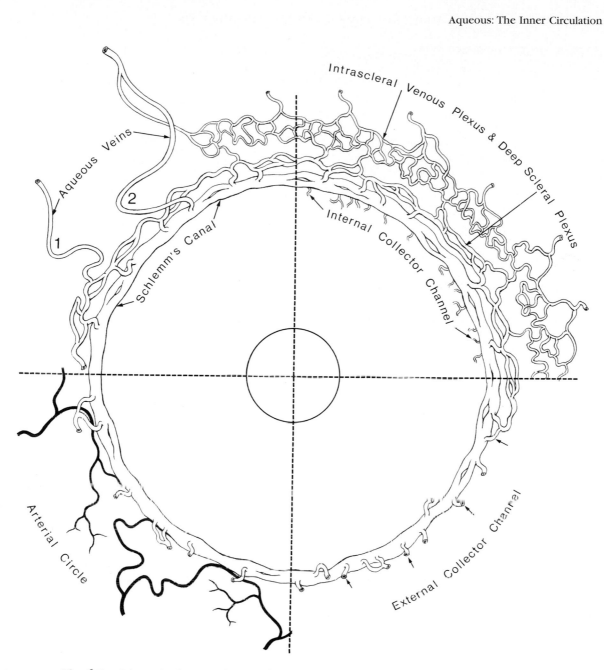

Fig. 6-5   Schematic drawing showing the circular course and related vessels of the canal of Schlemm. The canal divides into two or more portions intermittently. The drawing is divided into four portions by the dotted lines. The internal collector channels of Sondermann are labeled in the upper right sector as they extend into the trabecular meshwork. The external collector channels are seen in the upper and lower right sectors, arising from the canal and uniting with the deep intrascleral plexus or extending directly to the episcleral veins. The deep and intrascleral venous plexuses are external to the canal. In the upper left sector an aqueous vein *(1)* arises from the deep scleral plexus and another *(2)* arises from Schlemm's canal and runs directly to the episcleral venous plexus. External collector veins are seen to arise from the canal and join the deep scleral plexus. In the lower left sector, the arteries of the deep sclera are seen to be in close relation to the canal of Schlemm. (From Hogan MA, Alvarado J, Weddell J: *Histology of the human eye*, Philadelphia, 1971, WB Saunders.)

oval in cross section, 350 to 500 μ in meridional diameter, by 5 to 30 μ in width. In some areas, it branches into two or three channels. Schlemm's canal is lined by an endothelium. The inward aspect of Schlemm's canal, adjacent to the trabecular meshwork, is lined by a spe-cialized endothelium that constitutes the greatest resistance to aqueous outflow. These cells are large, 50 μ in diameter, and very thin, with a discontinuous basement membrane. The exact mechanism of resistance is not fully understood.

> ### MAJOR POINTS
>
> The aqueous fluid functions as a clear, colorless substitute for blood and nourishes the avascular cornea and lens.
>
> Aqueous fluid is a modified ultrafiltrate of blood plasma. The epithelial layers of the ciliary body take up blood plasma from the ciliary capillaries and secrete glucose, ions, and other substances into the posterior chamber.
>
> The aqueous fluid leaves the posterior chamber through the pupil, entering the anterior chamber.
>
> The trabecular meshwork lies between Schwalbe's line at the termination of Descemet's membrane and the scleral spur, although the most inward portion of the meshwork inserts into the ciliary body directly.
>
> The aqueous exits the eye through the trabecular meshwork into Schlemm's canal, from which it is returned to the vascular circulation. The site of resistance to aqueous outflow is believed to lie in the juxtacanalicular cells on the inner aspect of Schlemm's canal.
>
> Some of the aqueous fluid enters the space between ciliary body and sclera, bypassing Schlemm's canal. This is called uveoscleral outflow.

The internal collector channels of Sondermann are now thought not to exist per se, but rather to be simply outpouchings of Schlemm's canal that increase its surface area.

Schlemm's canal in turn is connected to the external collector channels that surround it. The aqueous mixes with blood here and enters the deep scleral plexus of veins. Thus the aqueous rejoins the blood circulation. The pressure differential between the venous circulation and Schlemm's canal is minimal; sometimes blood backs up and is visible within the canal.

Uveoscleral Outflow

A portion of the aqueous bypasses Schlemm's canal and enters the ciliary body and into the space between ciliary body and sclera, exiting the eye through the sclera. In primates, up to 35% of the aqueous exits in this manner, although clinical estimates in humans are uncertain. However, this portion of aqueous drainage is not subject to the resistance encountered in Schlemm's canal.

SUGGESTED READINGS

Anderson DR: Scanning electron microscopy of primate trabecular meshwork, *Am J Ophthalmol* 71:90-101, 1971.

Camras CB, Yablonski ME, Toris CB: The flow of aqueous humor. In Van Buskirk EM, Shields MB, editors: *100 years of glaucoma research,* pp 7-19, Philadelphia, 1997, Lippincott Raven.

Marshall GE, Konstas AGP, Lee WR: Immunogold ultrastructural localization of collagens in the aged human outflow system, *Ophthalmology* 98:692-700, 1991.

Morrison JC, Van Buskirk EM: Ciliary process microvasculature of the primate eye, *Am J Ophthalmol* 97:372-383, 1984.

Murphy CG, Yun AJ, Newsome DA, Alvarado JA: Localization of extracellular proteins of the human trabecular meshwork by indirect immunofluorescence, *Am J Ophthalmol* 104:33-43, 1987.

Tripathi BJ, Tripathi RC: Neural crest origin of human trabecular meshwork and its implications for the pathogenesis of glaucoma, *Am J Ophthalmol* 107:583-590, 1989.

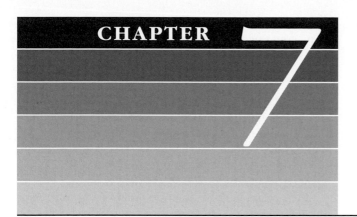

Uveal Tract: The Pigmented Layer

How is the entry of light into the eye controlled? The eye requires light to function, but light should enter in only one place and under controlled conditions to ensure proper function. The uveal tract is the pigmented layer of the eye.

But the uveal tract has other functions. Anteriorly it is clinically visible as the constantly moving iris. The iris in turn is continuous with the ciliary body, which controls accommodation and is also responsible for aqueous fluid synthesis. Posteriorly, the ciliary body joins with the bulk of the uveal tract, the choroid, which is concerned with retinal nutrition.

The uveal tract has two structural portions, the double-layered neuroepithelium with its regional variations and the stroma, derived from neural crest. Because at least one layer of the neuroectoderm is densely pigmented at any location in the uveal tract, the eye is "light-tight," allowing light to enter only through the pupil. Moreover, the pigmentation of the neuroectoderm is independent of racial or familial pigmentation or lack thereof—only albinos lack pigmentation of the neuroectoderm (and this lack of pigmentation leads to other abnormalities).

IRIS

The iris covers most of the anterior aspect of the lens surface. Its major function is to control light entering the eye. At 0.6 mm, it is thickest at the collarette, the area about 1.5 mm from the pupil margin. The pupil is the opening that occupies the approximate center of the iris. It is round in primates, but not necessarily in other species.

Pupil

Given the vast range over which the eye must function—from near-total darkness on a moonless night to the intense sunlight of a cloudless day at the beach—controlling entry of light is a considerable challenge. This challenge is met by the two smooth muscles of the iris, each innervated by one of the two opposing aspects of the autonomic nervous system, the parasympathetic and the sympathetic systems.

These two systems are constantly in a state of dynamic opposition. We see this readily when we examine any normal person, particularly with the magnification afforded by the slit lamp. Even with constant illumination, with the subject's eye fixated on a target, the iris moves slightly, dilating and constricting in turn, normally by less than 1 mm in diameter. This variation in pupil size is called *hippus,* the Greek word for horse. The observer who gave this name was struck by this undulating alteration, which called to mind the rhythmic galloping of a horse.

The parasympathetic innervation of the iris is derived from the autonomic portion of cranial nerve III. This portion synapses in the ciliary ganglion in the orbit. The postsynaptic fibers enter the eye with the short ciliary nerves.

The sympathetic innervation is derived from the cervical sympathetic chain. Fibers synapse at the superior cervical ganglion and then travel up with the internal carotid artery before entering the orbit along with the ophthalmic nerve. The postganglionic fibers proceed anteriorly as part of the long posterior ciliary nerves that enter the sclera at 3 and 9 o'clock.

Structure

Epithelial layers No matter what the level of pigmentation of the stroma, the posterior surface of the iris is always highly pigmented (Fig. 7-1). This helps maintain the "light-tight" characteristic of the globe. The posterior layer of epithelium is completely pigmented and is called the iris pigment epithelium. It is derived from the inner layer of the optic cup and thus is continuous with the nonpigmented epithelium of the ciliary body. These cells are cuboidal, with the basement membrane posterior. Numerous melanosomes, both spherical and elongated, fill the cytoplasm. All of these melanosomes are mature and thus are densely and homogeneously pigmented. Tight junctions, or desmosomes, join the posterior cells together and also join the posterior layer of cells to the cells of the anterior layer.

The anterior layer is called the dilator muscle, even though only a portion of the cell (the basal portion, facing anteriorly) is differentiated into smooth muscle. The apical portion of the cell contains the nucleus and melanosomes similar to those of the posterior layer. By light microscopy, the cell boundaries of the pigmented portions of the two cell layers cannot be discerned; bleaching or electron microscopy is necessary to disclose the cellular arrangement.

The dilator muscle lines essentially the entire iris stroma except at the pupil. The individual cells are joined together by multiple desmosomes, and thus the muscle can contract as a unit. Histologically, the muscle is seen as an eosinophilic band just anterior to the dense pigmentation of the neuroepithelium, because this portion of the cell is not pigmented.

When we perform a slit lamp examination, no matter what color the iris stroma is, we see a rim of darkly pigmented cells at the pupil margin. This is where the anterior neuroectodermal layer becomes continuous with the posterior layer (Fig. 7-2).

The sphincter muscle forms a circle surrounding the pupil and is separate from the double neuroepithelial layer posterior to it (Fig. 7-3). This separation from the neuroectoderm occurs early in embryogenesis. Histologically and ultrastructurally it is composed of typical smooth muscle cells. These connect via thin muscular strands to iris stroma and to the dilator muscle.

Stroma The iris stroma is a loose, open complex of fibrocytes, collagen, melanocytes, blood vessels, and nerves (Fig. 7-4). There is no anterior boundary as such; rather, the anterior surface is open, with crypts, as we see clinically and especially well in a light-colored eye. The melanocytes are present throughout the stroma, although they are more clustered along the anterior surface (Fig. 7-5). This clustering is especially prominent in dark irises, such that clinically they have a smoother appearing surface, with less prominent crypts. Melanin, mainly contained within the melanocytes, is responsible for iris color. Blue color is a phenomenon of light diffraction and scatter by collagen fibers; there is no blue pigment. The iris color seems independent of the number of melanocytes, but the number of melanosomes does differ, with increasing number in darker-colored irises. Plump, round clump cells are also present, especially at deeper layers of the stroma. They are phagocytic and consume but do not produce melanin.

The stroma contains the blood vessels of the iris. The arterioles originate and branch radially from the major arterial circle of the iris (which, despite its name, is actually located in anterior ciliary body) and proceed centrally toward the pupil. The blood vessels macroscopically have a somewhat spiral configuration. They are concentrically arranged near the pupil.

The major arterial circle receives its blood supply from the seven anterior ciliary arteries, as well as from anterior branches from the two long posterior ciliary arteries. In addition to supplying the iris and ciliary body, these vessels also make contributions to the choriocapillaris anteriorly.

A notable microscopic feature of the iris arterioles is their very thick walls. These thick vessel walls are evident even in children and do not indicate arteriosclerosis. Instead, they are the result of the constant motion of the iris, in turn stretching and kinking the vessels.

CILIARY BODY

The ciliary body is roughly triangular shaped when seen in cross section. From its anterior insertion at the scleral spur back to the ora serrata, it measures about 6 to 6.5 mm. It can be divided into two regions, the pars plicata, or pleated part, and the pars plana, or flat part. The pars plicata is about 2 mm from anterior to posterior and consists of about 70 ciliary processes. These provide considerable surface area for secretion of aqueous fluid.

The pars plana, which is about 4 to 4.5 mm, is the area where entry into the posterior portion of the eye is safest, with least disruption of other intraocular structures.

Structure

Epithelial layers The two layers of the neuroectoderm are readily distinguishable in the region of the ciliary body (Fig. 7-6). The inner layer, the nonpigmented epithelium, is a monolayer of cuboidal cells continuous with the iris pigment epithelium anteriorly and the sensory retina posteriorly (Box 7-1). The outer layer, the pigment epithelium, is continuous anteriorly with the dilator muscle of the iris and with the retinal pigment

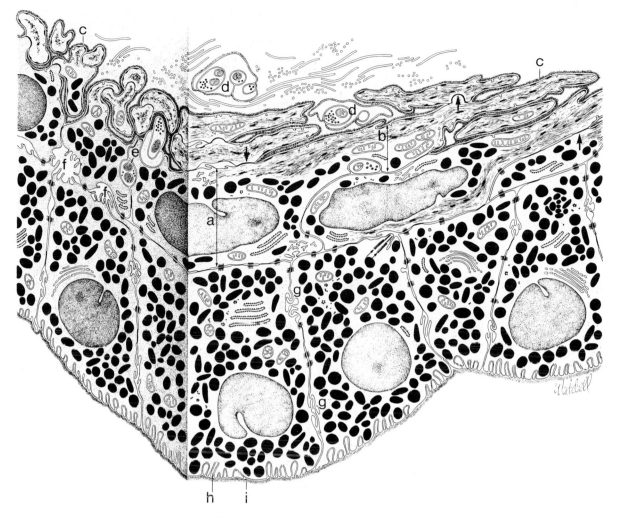

Fig. 7-1   Posterior epithelial layers. The anterior iris epithelium has two morphologically distinct portions: an apical epithelial portion *(a)* and a basal muscular portion *(b)*. The cytoplasm of the basal portion is filled with myofibrils and a moderate number of mitochondria. The tonguelike muscular processes overlap each other, creating three to five layers. Tight junctions *(arrows)* like those in the sphincter muscle are found between the dilator muscle cells. A basement membrane *(c)* surrounds the muscle processes. Unmyelinated nerves and their associated Schwann cells *(d)* as well as a few naked axons innervate the muscle. The axon at *(e)* is in close contact with the anterior epithelium, being separated from it by a space measuring 200 Å in width. The cytoplasm of the epithelial portions contains cell organelles, melanin granules, the nucleus, and bundles of myofilaments. Most of the intercellular junctions present here are maculae occludentes and only a few desmosomes are present; desmosomes are not found in the muscular portion. The apical surface of the anterior epithelium is contiguous with that of the posterior epithelium. Desmosomes and tight junctions join the two layers, but there are some areas of separation *(f)* between the cells. The spaces so formed are filled with microvilli, and an occasional cilium is also found here *(double arrows)*. The posterior pigmented iris epithelium shows lateral interdigitations *(g)* and areas of infolding along its basal surface *(h)*. A typical basement membrane is also found on the basal side *(i)*. Numerous tight junctions and desmosomes occur along the lateral and apical walls. The cytoplasm of this epithelium has numerous melanin granules measuring around 0.8 μm in cross-section and up to 2.5 μm in length. Stacks of cisternae of the rough-surfaced endoplasmic reticulum, clustered unattached ribosomes, mitochondria, and a Golgi apparatus are commonly observed. (From Hogan MA, Alvarado J, Weddell J: *Histology of the human eye,* Philadelphia, 1971, WB Saunders.)

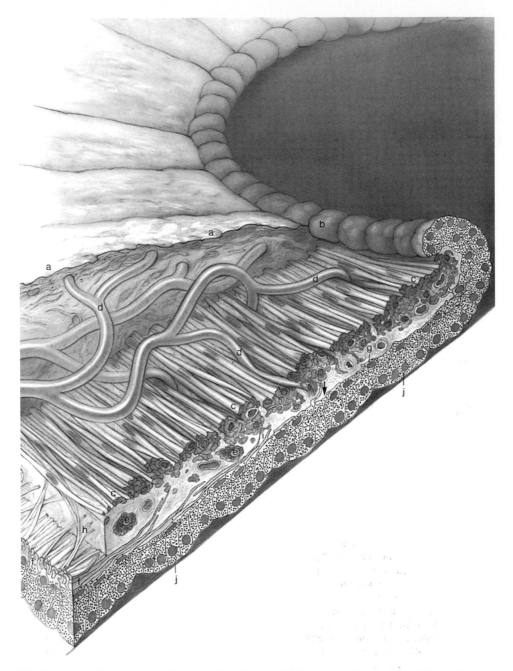

Fig. 7-2   Pupillary portion of the iris. The dense, cellular anterior border layer *(a)* terminates at the pigment ruff *(b)* in the pupillary margin. The sphincter muscle is at *(c)*. The arcades *(d)* from the minor circle extend toward the pupil and through the sphincter muscle. The sphincter muscle and the iris epithelium are close to each other at the pupillary margin. Capillaries, nerves, melanocytes, and clump cells *(e)* are found within and around the muscle. The three to five layers of dilator muscle *(f)* gradually diminish in number until they terminate behind the midportion of the sphincter muscle *(arrow),* leaving low, cuboidal epithelial cells *(g)* to form the anterior epithelium to the pupillary margin. Spurlike extensions from the dilator muscle form Michel's spur *(h)* and Fuchs' spur *(i),* which extend anteriorly to blend with the sphincter muscle. The posterior epithelium *(j)* is formed by tall columnar cells with basally located nuclei. Its apical surface is contiguous with the apical surface of the anterior epithelium. (From Hogan MA, Alvarado J, Weddell J: *Histology of the human eye,* Philadelphia, 1971, WB Saunders.)

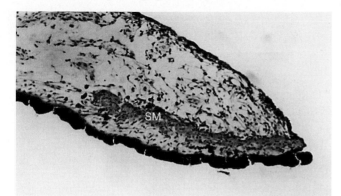

Fig. 7-3   Iris at the papillary margin. The sphincter muscle (SM) is a dense band anterior to the pigment epithelium. Hematoxylin and eosin, ×80. (See color plate.)

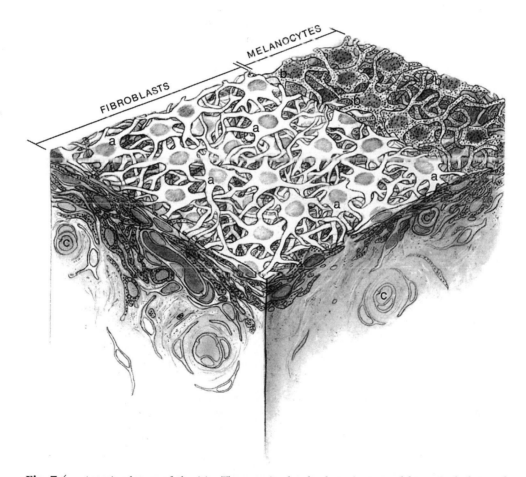

Fig. 7-4   Anterior layers of the iris. The anterior border layer is covered by a single layer of fibroblasts *(a)* whose long, branching processes interconnect with each other. The branching processes of the fibroblasts form openings of various sizes on the iris surface. Beneath the layer of fibroblasts is a fairly dense aggregation of melanocytes and a few fibroblasts. The superficial layer of fibroblasts has been removed at *b* to show these cells. The number of cells in the anterior border layer is greater than the number in the underlying stroma. The iris stroma contains a number of capillaries *(c),* which sometimes are quite close to the surface. (From Hogan MA, Alvarado J, Weddell J: *Histology of the human eye,* Philadelphia, 1971, WB Saunders.)

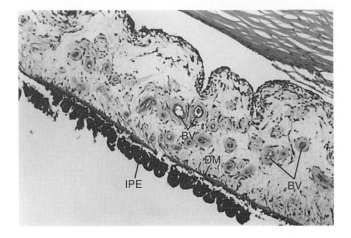

Fig. 7-5 The iris. The anterior margin has more dense pigmentation but is nevertheless an open meshwork. Blood vessels *(BV)* with thick walls are prominent. Just anterior to the iris pigment epithelium *(IPE)* is a thin eosinophilic band, the dilator muscle *(DM)*. Hematoxylin and eosin, ×80. (See color plate.)

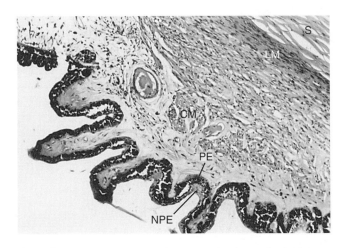

Fig. 7-6 The ciliary body. The longitudinal muscle *(LM)* is apposed to the sclera *(S)*. More internally is the circular muscle *(CM)*. The ciliary processes are covered by a double epithelial layer, the outer pigmented epithelium *(PE)* and inner nonpigmented epithelium *(NPE)*. Hematoxylin and eosin, ×80. (See color plate.)

epithelium posteriorly. Both of the ciliary epithelial layers are responsible for secreting the aqueous fluid.

Stroma The ciliary body stroma consists of melanocytes and fibrocytes along with smooth muscle and blood vessels (Fig. 7-7). Functionally, we can think of these as being two muscles, the outer longitudinal muscle and the inner circular muscle. However, the muscular structure forms a continuum, so that the fibers, as going from outward to inward, are longitudinally oriented, then more radial, and then finally circular. The radial muscle does not appear to have a specific function; it simply represents the transition zone. The ciliary muscles are

---

Box 7-1 Layers of the Neuroectoderm

INNER NEUROECTODERMAL LAYER
Iris pigment epithelium
Ciliary body nonpigment epithelium
Sensory retina

OUTER NEUROECTODERMAL LAYER
Iris dilator muscle
Ciliary body pigment epithelium
Retinal pigment epithelium

---

innervated by parasympathetic fibers that have synapsed in the ciliary ganglion and accompanied the third nerve forward into the eye.

The longitudinal muscle is attached anteriorly to the scleral spur. This is the most firm attachment of ciliary body to sclera, remaining inserted even when the remainder of the ciliary body is detached by a fluid effusion. Tension on the longitudinal muscle appears to open up the trabecular meshwork, facilitating aqueous fluid drainage.

The circular muscle is the innermost portion of muscle; it is located just external to the ciliary processes. Contraction of this muscle draws the ciliary body inward, relaxing the zonular fibers on the lens and allowing the lens to assume a more spherical shape.

CHOROID

The choroid is the posterior portion of the uveal tract, continuous with the ciliary body anteriorly, and terminating at the optic nerve posteriorly. Its purpose is to nourish the retina, and as a consequence, it is no surprise that the blood vessels are the most conspicuous aspect of the choroid (Fig. 7-8). When congested, they substantially thicken the choroidal parenchyma and give it a spongy consistency. In addition to the vessels, the choroid contains uveal melanocytes and scattered fibrocytes.

The blood supply of the uveal tract comes from several sources, although all are ultimately derived from the ophthalmic artery. Fifteen to 20 short posterior ciliary arteries enter through the sclera in the area adjacent to the optic nerve and supply the posterior aspect. They run in the suprachoroidal space, between choroid and sclera, for a short distance, then branch and extend anteriorly to approximately the equator.

The two long posterior ciliary arteries enter the sclera at the horizontal meridian posteriorly, proceeding anteriorly within the sclera to the ciliary body. They branch

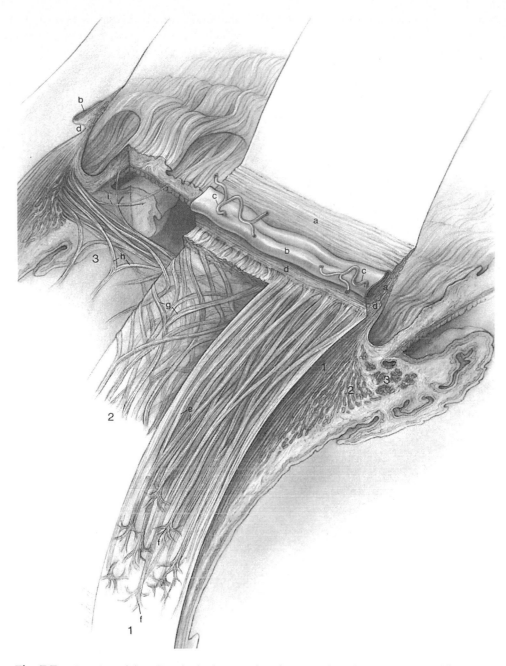

Fig. 7-7   Drawing of the ciliary body showing the ciliary muscle and its components. The cornea and sclera have been dissected away but the trabecular meshwork (a), Schlemm's canal (b), and two external collectors (c), as well as the scleral spur (d), have been left undisturbed. The three components of the ciliary muscle are shown separately, viewed from the outside, and sectioned meridionally. Section 1 shows the *longitudinal* ciliary muscle; in section 2 the longitudinal ciliary muscle has been dissected away to show the *radial* ciliary muscle; in section 3 only the innermost *circular* ciliary muscle is shown. According to Calasans (1953), the ciliary muscle originates in the ciliary tendon, which includes the scleral spur (d) and the adjacent connective tissue. The cells originate as paired V-shaped bundles. The *longitudinal* muscle forms long V-shaped trellises (e) which terminate in the epichoroidal stars (f). The arms of the V-shaped bundles formed by the *radial* muscle meet at wide angles (g) and terminate in the ciliary processes. The V-shaped bundles of the circular muscle originate at such distant points in the ciliary tendon that their arms meet at a very wide angle (h). The iridic portion is shown at (i) joining the circular muscle cells. (From Hogan MA, Alvarado J, Weddell J: *Histology of the human eye,* Philadelphia, 1971, WB Saunders.)

at about the level of the ora serrata and supply much of the anterior uveal circulation, but some branches also loop back into the anterior choroid.

The choroid is drained by means of the vortex veins. These are located just posterior to the equator and are clinically visible, particularly in blond fundi, as irregular star-shaped structures. Choroidal venules come together

and drain into a dilated structure, the ampulla, from which the vortex vein pierces the sclera and exits the eye. Although drawings typically show four of these, located superonasal, superotemporal, inferotemporal, and inferonasal, the number actually varies in different eyes, averaging about seven per eye; they are more numerous nasally.

Within the choroid itself, the largest vessels are closest to the sclera, whereas the layer with the smallest vessels is the choriocapillaris, the innermost layer. The choriocapillaris is a monolayer of interlacing capillaries and is distinctive for having the largest capillaries in the body, up to 20 μ in diameter in the macula and up to 50 μ peripherally. These vessels nourish the metabolically active retinal pigment epithelium and outer retina. The choroidal system is a high-flow, low-resistance system (Fig. 7-9). The density of the choriocapillaris decreases with age.

Although it appears anatomically that the capillaries of the choriocapillaris form a diffuse network throughout the choroid, it is evident both from postmortem studies and from fluorescein angiography that there are distinct filling patterns. In the posterior pole, the capillaries are arranged in a lobular pattern, with a feeding arteriole in the center of each lobule and several venules draining the lobule peripherally. The arterioles taper rapidly to form multiple capillaries, and this accounts for the high rate of blood flow through the capillary bed. This high flow rate appears to function at least in part as a heat-dissipating

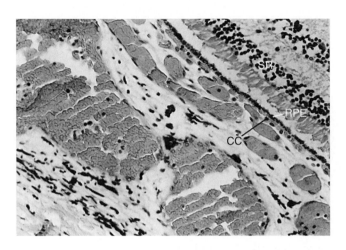

Fig. 7-8 The choroid with its large, prominent vessels. The sensory retina *(SR)* overlies the retinal pigmented epithelium *(RPE)*. Just beneath the pigment epithelium are the large capillaries of the choriocapillaris *(CC)*. Hematoxylin and eosin, ×80. (See color plate.)

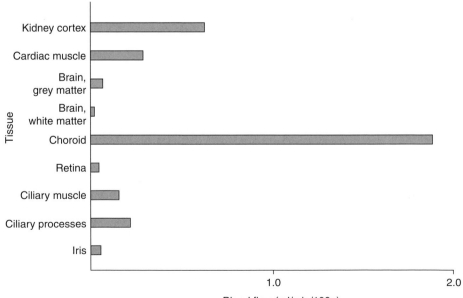

Fig. 7-9 Blood flow through tissues of monkey eye. Flow through other tissues is included for comparison. (Values for blood flow through ocular tissues from Alm et al, 1973. Values for extraocular tissues are taken from Folkow and Neil, 1971.) (From Hart WM, editor: *Adler's physiology of the eye,* ed 9, St Louis, 1992, Mosby.)

mechanism. There are also numerous arteriole-arteriole anastomoses, particularly in the posterior pole.

In the far periphery, the choroidal vessels are arranged more longitudinally, with the arteries and veins being more parallel, connected by capillaries in a manner suggesting a ladder. At the equator, the configuration is a transition between these two arrangements, a spindle configuration. In this region, the venules tend to be more central and the arterioles more peripheral.

The capillaries have fenestrations, or pores, which are most numerous on the inner aspect of the capillaries, toward the pigment epithelium. This allows diffusion of metabolites to and from the pigment epithelium and outer aspect of sensory retina. Ultrastructurally, these fenestrations consist of small circular areas 60 mm in diameter in the unit membrane of the capillary endothe-

lium (see Fig. 9-1). They appear to be focal fusions of the two unit membranes from either side of the cytoplasm, with no cytoplasm between. Like capillaries elsewhere, individual endothelial cells are joined together by tight junctions, or zonulae occludentes.

The choroid is innervated by the short posterior ciliary nerves. These enter and travel with the short posterior ciliary arteries. They remain myelinated for a short distance within the eye and then become unmyelinated. They appear to supply sympathetic innervation to the blood vessels.

The long posterior ciliary nerves enter at the horizontal meridians, at 3 and 9 o'clock, along with the long posterior ciliary arteries. The nerves travel in the suprachoroidal space, between choroid and sclera, and remain myelinated until arriving in the ciliary body.

The choroidal melanocytes are derived from neural crest. They are star-shaped and have many long delicate processes. They contain numerous small round to oval melanosomes and retain the ability to synthesize melanin throughout life. Other cells present in the choroid include scattered fibrocytes.

The choroid, like the ciliary body, is attached to the sclera by means of long, interconnecting collagen fibers, called the lamina fusca. Within this suprachoroidea are melanocytes and nerve plexuses. The attachments between choroid and sclera are essentially perpendicular posteriorly, keeping the choroid relatively tightly bound, but become more obliquely oriented anteriorly. Thus suprachoroidal fluid preferentially collects anteriorly, no matter where the stimulus is actually located.

MAJOR POINTS

The entire uveal tract makes the eye "light-tight," allowing light to enter only through the pupil.

Throughout the uvea, at least one layer of the neuroepithelium is densely pigmented.

Neuroepithelial pigmentation is dense, regardless of racial or familial background, whereas neural crest (uveal stromal) pigmentation varies according to racial and genetic factors.

Parasympathetic innervation to the sphincter causes pupillary constriction, whereas sympathetic innervation to the iris dilator muscle widens the pupil.

The iris dilator and sphincter muscles both arise from the anterior layer of the neuroepithelium.

There is no epithelial layer on the anterior surface of the iris; rather, it is an open mesh of fibrocytes and melanocytes.

The iris arterioles normally have remarkably thick walls, the result of the constant motion of the iris.

The longitudinal muscle of the ciliary body attaches anteriorly to the scleral spur. This is the strongest attachment between ciliary body and sclera. It receives parasympathetic innervation.

The circular muscle of the ciliary body controls accommodation. Stimulation by it parasympathetic innervation causes contraction, allowing the zonules to relax and the lens to become more spherical.

The choroid underlies the retina and is responsible for nutrition to the retinal pigment epithelium and outer aspect of sensory retina. The capillaries of the choriocapillaris are the largest in the human body.

The ciliary body and choroid are connected to the sclera via long collagen fibers, called the lamina fusca. These attachments are more perpendicular posteriorly but more oblique anteriorly. Thus fluid collecting between uvea and sclera tends to collect anteriorly.

SUGGESTED READINGS

Imesch PD, Bindley CD, Khademian Z, et al: Melanocytes and iris color: electron microscopic findings, *Arch Ophthalmol* 114:443-447, 1996.

Lim MC, Bateman JB, Glasgow BJ: Vortex vein exit sites: scleral coordinates, *Ophthalmology* 102:942-946, 1995.

McLeod DS, Lutty GA: High-resolution histologic analysis of the human choroidal vasculature, *Invest Ophthalmol Vis Sci* 35: 3799-3811, 1994.

Parver LM, Auker C, Carpenter DO: Choroidal blood flow as a heat dissipating mechanism in the macula, *Am J Ophthalmol* 89:641-646, 1980.

Smith-Thomas L, Richardson P, Thody AJ, et al: Human ocular melanocytes and retinal pigment epithelial cells differ in their melanogenic properties *in vivo* and *in vitro, Curr Eye Res* 15:1079-1091, 1996.

Spitznas M, Reale E: Fracture faces of fenestrations and junctions of endothelial cells in human choroidal vessels, *Invest Ophthalmol* 14:98-107, 1975.

Wilkerson CL, Syed NA, Fisher MR, et al: Melanocytes and iris color: light microscopic findings, *Arch Ophthalmol* 114: 437-442, 1996.

Yoneya S, Tso MO: Angioarchitecture of the human choroid, *Arch Ophthalmol* 105:681-687, 1987.

CHAPTER 8

Lens and Accommodation

How is light focused on the retina? In addition, how can the focus be varied for the differing distances under which the eye must function? The lens power is about 20 diopters, about one-third of the total focusing power of the eye. More notably, the lens in younger persons is capable of changing shape, so that the eye can focus near and at a distance.

LENS STRUCTURE

The lens is remarkable for being an "inside-out" structure. During embryonic development, the lens, which originates from the surface ectoderm, invaginates toward the optic cup and then separates and migrates posteriorly. Thus the basement membrane is peripheral, and the cells are enclosed within. This basement membrane is what we refer to clinically as the lens capsule.

The lens has no blood supply and no innervation. As a living tissue, it depends on the circulating aqueous fluid for nutrition.

The lens is about 35% protein, a protein content about twice as high as that in other living tissues. Thus its transparency is perhaps even more remarkable, and the mechanism of this transparency is not well understood. The lens crystallins account for nearly all the protein. The crystallins were once thought to be unique to the lens,

but, in fact, they are widely distributed throughout other body tissues.

Lens Capsule

The capsule varies in thickness regionally (Fig. 8-1). Anteriorly, it is uniform and 12 to 21 μ thick. Immediately posterior to the capsule is a single layer of epithelial cells (Fig. 8-2). The capsule thins slightly as it goes around the equator to about 9 to 17 μ. Paracentrally, it again thickens. Here the lens is attached to the secondary (adult) vitreous by Wieger's ligament, the hyalocapsular ligament. Wieger's ligament is not a true ligament, but is simply a circular area of adhesion about 8 mm in diameter, which corresponds to the most anterior aspect of Cloquet's canal, the remnant of the primary vitreous. This adhesion is strong in infants and children, but weak or nonexistent in older persons. At the posterior pole, the capsule is thinnest, only 2 to 9 μ (Fig. 8-3). The capsule is a typical basement membrane, composed of type IV collagen.

The lens zonules merge with the lens capsule, both anteriorly and posteriorly.

Lens Epithelium

Anteriorly, the lens epithelial cells remain as a low cuboidal, single layer of cells just beneath the anterior capsule. Metabolic activity is low, as disclosed by the sparse organelles seen by electron microscopy. The epithelium continues to proliferate very slowly throughout life; this proliferation takes place in the paracentral germinative zone. The cells migrate more peripherally to the equator, where they move inward, gradually lose their nuclei, and become new lens fibers.

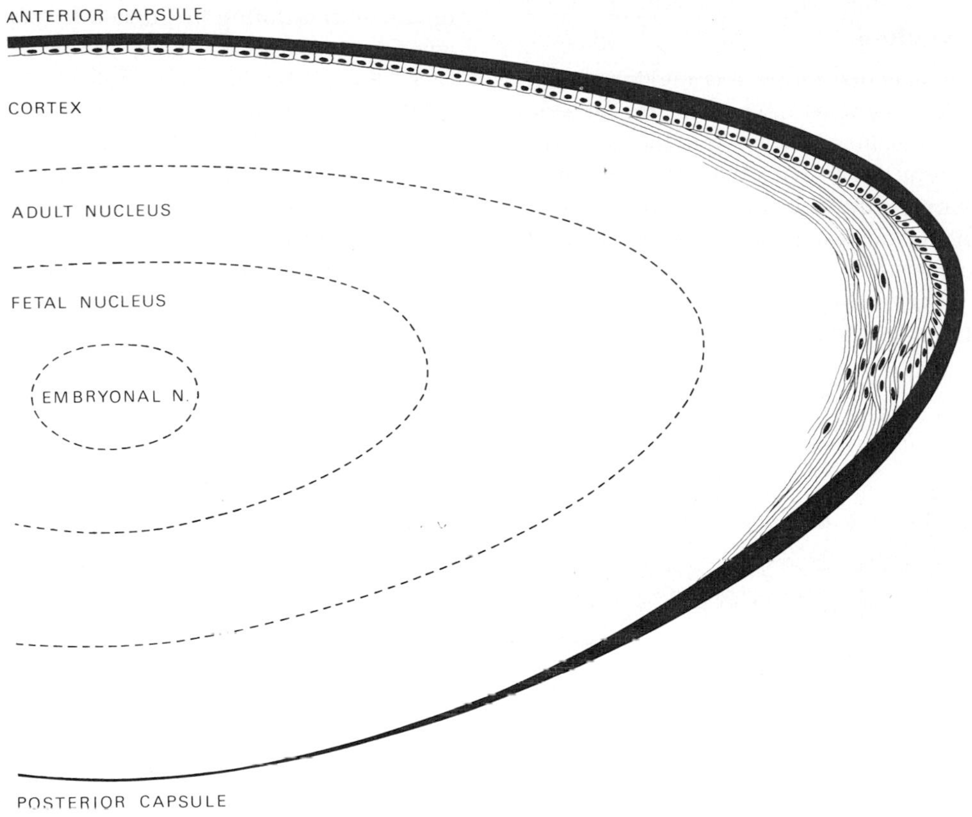

ANTERIOR CAPSULE

CORTEX

ADULT NUCLEUS

FETAL NUCLEUS

EMBRYONAL N.

POSTERIOR CAPSULE

Fig. 8-1   Schematic representation of the adult lens, showing the nuclear zones, epithelium, and capsule. The thickness of the lens capsule in various zones is shown. (From Hogan MA, Alvarado J, Weddell J: *Histology of the human eye,* Philadelphia, 1971, WB Saunders.)

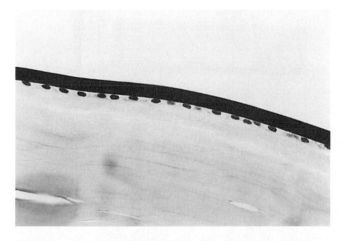

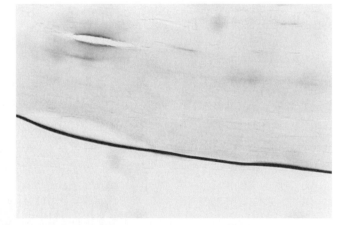

Fig. 8-2   High-power view of the anterior lens capsule and epithelium immediately beneath. The anterior cortex appears structureless. Periodic acid-Schiff, ×625.

Fig. 8-3   High-power view of the posterior lens capsule at the same magnification as that for Fig. 8-2. Periodic acid-Schiff, ×625.

Cortex and Nucleus

When the lens vesicle first forms, it is a hollow sphere of cells with the basement membrane on the outside. The anterior cells remain cuboidal, but the posterior cells elongate to form fibers that obliterate the central space. These constitute the primary lens fibers, which form the embryonal nucleus. Subsequent proliferation gives rise to secondary lens fibers.

As the cells elongate, they migrate inward, forming the fetal and adult nuclei and finally the cortex. The fetal nucleus forms during the remainder of gestation, and the adult nucleus forms during youth. The boundaries of these nuclei can be seen clinically in young adults as bright bands, giving the optical cross section of the lens the appearance of an onion. These boundaries are areas where growth is evidently altered or temporarily slowed, but they cannot be seen histologically, and their exact nature remains unknown.

Individual lens fibers extend in a C shape from anterior to posterior, with the disintegrating nucleus in the middle, in the equatorial region. In cross section, they

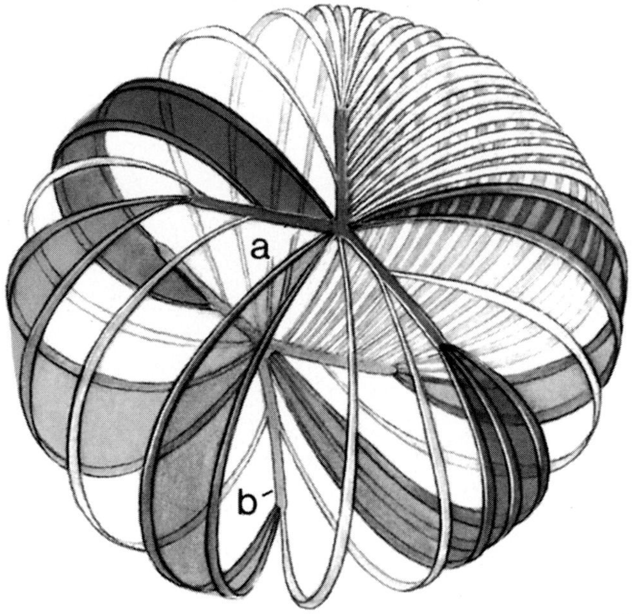

Fig. 8-4 Embryonal and adult lens show the sutures and arrangement of the lens cells. **A,** Drawing of the embryonal nucleus. The anterior Y suture is at *a* and the posterior at *b*. The lens cells are depicted as wide, colored bands. Those cells that attach to the tips of the Y sutures at one pole of the lens attach to the fork of the Y at the opposite pole. It can be seen if the lens cell attaches to the tip of a Y suture anteriorly or its distance from the equator is shorter at the pole of the lens. **B,** Adult lens cortex. The anterior and posterior organization of the sutures is more complex. Those lens cells that arise from the tip of a branch of the suture insert farther anteriorly or posteriorly into a fork at the posterior pole. This arrangement conserves the shape of the lens. This drawing shows the suture to lie in a single plane for pictorial reasons, but it should be remembered that it extends throughout the thickness of the cortex and nucleus to the level of the Y sutures in the embryonal nucleus. (From Hogan MA, Alvarado J, Weddell J: *Histology of the human eye,* Philadelphia, 1971, WB Saunders.) (See color plate.)

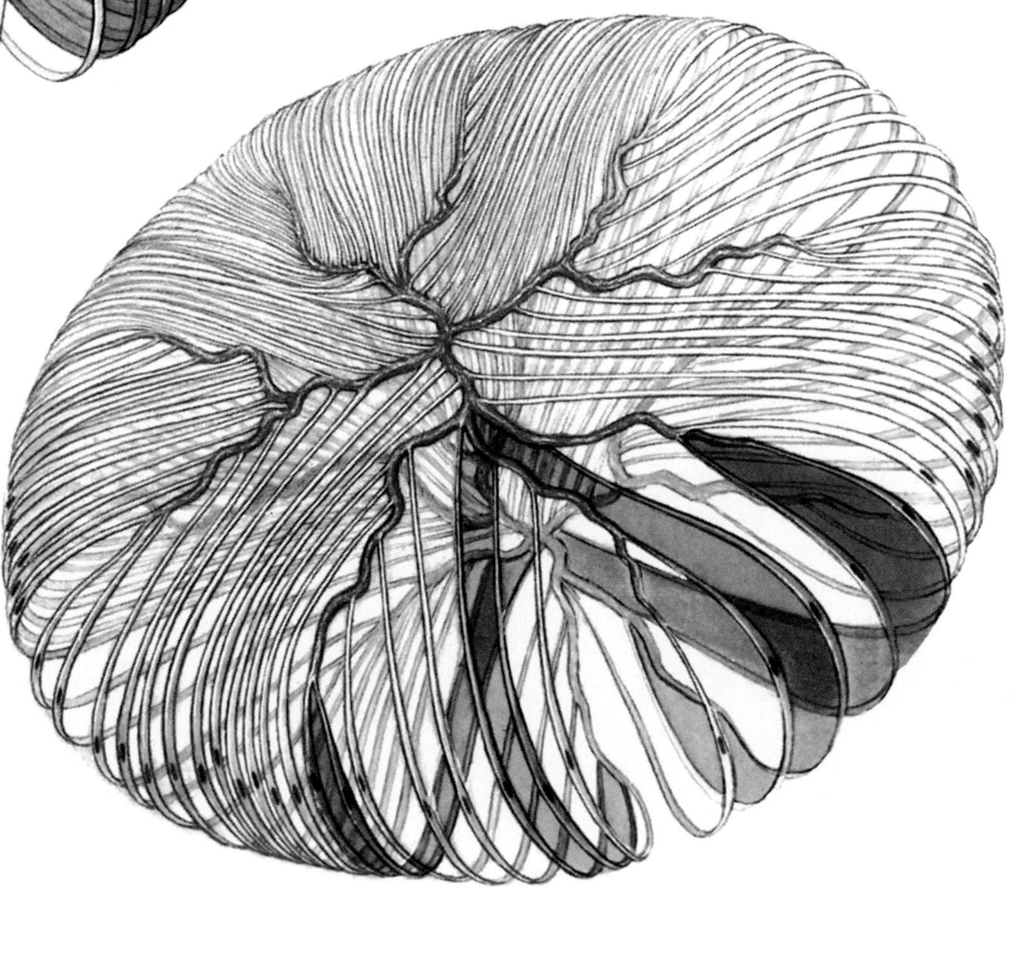

have a flattened hexagonal shape. Obviously, the fibers cannot all come together in one place. In the fetal nucleus, the anterior and posterior ends of the fibers are arranged in such a way that they form Y sutures (Fig. 8-4). The Y is upright anteriorly but inverted posteriorly. The Y sutures are most easily seen in young persons. With succeeding layers of fibers, the Y sutures are obscured,

and the fiber junctions take on a more dendritic appearance.

The cortex develops slowly throughout life. The lens fibers of the cortex are the most peripheral of the lens. The cortical cells have a bland cytoplasm with few organelles. Cortical and nuclear cells are tightly bound to each other by means of "ball and socket" joints (Fig. 8-5).

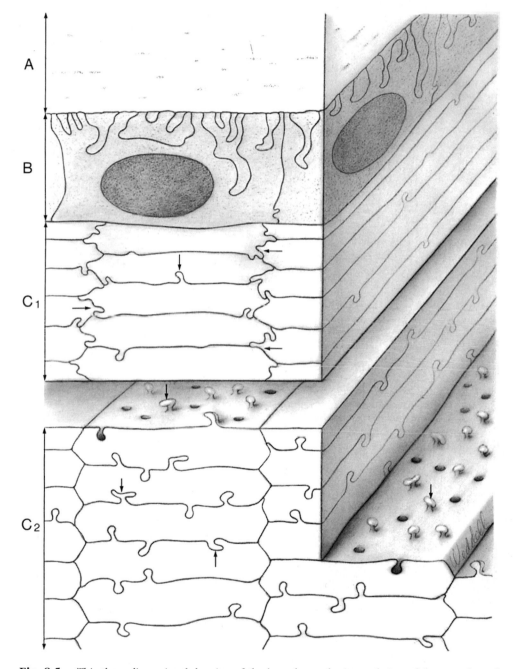

Fig. 8-5   This three-dimensional drawing of the lens shows the interrelation of the capsule and underlying lens cells. The capsule is at *A* and shows inclusion of fine filamentous material. The anterior lens epithelium *(B)* shows interdigitation of its basal surface with adjacent hexagonal ends as well as along their edges *(C₁) (arrows)*. The deeper cortical cells *(C₂)* also show a tongue-and-groove type of interdigitation along their long sides *(arrows),* but the interlocking is absent at the short ends. (From Hogan MA, Alvarado J, Weddell J: *Histology of the human eye,* Philadelphia, 1971, WB Saunders.)

Zonules

The lens is held in its central location by hundreds of zonules. These zonules attach to the anterior and posterior lens capsule and appear to originate from the ciliary body, not only between the processes of the pars plicata but also from pars plana and even from the peripheral retina.

During embryonic life, the developing lens is nourished by the hyaloid system, the primary vitreous. The hyaloid artery arborizes behind the lens, forming the tunica vasculosa lentis. This system is most developed by the end of the third fetal month and then begins to atrophy as the secondary vitreous forms, displacing the primary vitreous centrally. By this time, the secondary vitreous surrounds the equator of the lens, but as the neuroectoderm of the optic cup continues to advance forward and the ciliary body and iris develop, the secondary vitreous is displaced posteriorly. The tertiary vitreous, another term for the zonules, begins to develop after the 12th gestational week, originating from the nonpigmented ciliary epithelium and advancing centrally to the lens capsule.

No collagen is present in the zonules. Instead, the zonules are aggregates of elastic fibers, composed of fibrillin, a glycoprotein rich in the amino acid cysteine.

Interestingly, the zonules appear to advance centrally on the anterior capsule with increasing age. Thus the width of zonule-free anterior capsule is more than 8 mm in young adults but declines to only 6 mm or less in older individuals.

The Circular Muscle

The circular muscle of the ciliary body controls accommodation. This muscle is the innermost of the ciliary body, located just external to the ciliary processes (see Figs. 7-6 and 7-7). Like any circular muscle, when it contracts, the circle becomes smaller. Concomitantly, the muscle moves inward to a somewhat more central position in the eye.

In the relaxed state, the lens is passively stretched by the zonules. In the emmetropic eye, this allows the focus of parallel light rays on the retina.

Accommodation is under parasympathetic control. With accommodation, three things happen: the pupil constricts, the eyes both move medially through contraction of both medial recti, and the circular muscle contracts, moving more centrally. In turn, the tension on the zonules is relaxed, and the lens, which if left to its own devices would rather be spherical, is allowed to approach this state. As determined through clinical measurements, most of the change in lens shape takes place

> ### MAJOR POINTS
>
> The lens originates from surface ectoderm. It is an "inside out" structure with basement membrane (lens capsule) outside and epithelium inside.
>
> The capsule is thickest anteriorly and thinnest at the posterior pole.
>
> The lens is avascular living tissue; its nutritional needs are supplied by the aqueous fluid.
>
> The lens epithelium anteriorly is a single layer of low cuboidal cells. The germinative area for new lens fibers lies in the anterior paracentral area. New fibers elongate anteriorly and posteriorly, lose their nuclei, and are pushed centrally as more fibers are formed. The lens slowly grows throughout life.
>
> The embryonal nucleus is the most central and deep nucleus. More peripheral fibers form the fetal and adult nuclei; the most peripheral form the cortex. The fibers are joined by ball-and-socket joints.
>
> Zonules, the tertiary vitreous, suspend the lens and passively stretch it. Contraction of the circular muscle of the ciliary body relaxes tension on the zonules, allowing the lens to become more spherical and increasing its plus power. The distensibility of the lens is lost with age.

posteriorly. This more spherical shape increases the plus power of the lens, allowing focusing of the divergent rays of near objects.

With age, as the lens hardens and becomes less distensible, accommodation is lost. At birth, the accommodative amplitude is 14 diopters or more; throughout life it gradually decreases, resulting in presbyopia in the 40s.

SUGGESTED READING

Apple DJ, Lim ES, Morgan RC, et al: Preparation and study of human eyes obtained postmortem with the Miyake posterior photographic technique, *Ophthalmology* 97:810-816, 1990.

Glasser A, Kaufman PL: The mechanism of accommodation in primates, *Ophthalmology* 106:863-872, 1999.

Hamming NA, Apple DJ, Gieser DK, Vygantas CM: Ultrastructure of the hyaloid vasculature in primates, *Invest Ophthalmol Vis Sci* 16:408-415, 1977.

Pavlin CJ, Buys YM, Pathmanathan T: Imaging zonular abnormalities using ultrasound biomicroscopy, *Arch Ophthalmol* 116:854-857, 1998.

Sakabe I, Oshika T, Lim SJ, Apple DJ: Anterior shift of zonular insertion onto the anterior surface of human crystalline lens with age, *Ophthalmology* 105:295-299, 1998.

Streeten B: The nature of the ocular zonule, *Trans Am Ophthalmol Soc* 80:823-854, 1982.

Retina and Optic Nerve: How We See

How do we actually see? For any stimulus—be it touch, pain, heat, cold, light, or sound—to be interpreted by the brain, the organism must first convert it into neural impulses that are then channeled to the brain along an afferent pathway. The retina, therefore, acts as the receptacle for the incoming light stimulus. But it does more; the retina begins the process of modulating the stimuli even before sending them on to the brain. The retina and optic nerve should therefore be thought of as a continuum, because anatomically they are connected, and they are both part of the central nervous system. (We should note also that all stimuli to the retina are interpreted as light. Thus the retina feels no pain. Traction or pressure on the retina is interpreted as sparks of light.)

A potential source of confusion is just how the term "retina" is used. Anatomically the retina includes the retinal pigment epithelium, but clinically, the retina usually means the sensory retina, excluding the pigment epithelium.

The retina is a wonderfully complicated structure. However, even at low-power magnification, it shows a striking order, with layers of nuclei separated by layers of nonnuclear material.

RETINAL PIGMENT EPITHELIUM

The retinal pigment epithelium remains a monolayer, under normal conditions, throughout embryogenesis and postnatal life. By light microscopy there appears to be little difference between this and its contiguous layer, the ciliary body pigment epithelium. However, ultrastructurally, major differences are apparent.

The retinal pigment epithelium, in concert with the photoreceptors, constitutes one of the most metabolically active tissues in the body. The retinal pigment epithelial cells are responsible for metabolizing the shed outer segments of the photoreceptors, and their structure reflects this function (Fig. 9-1). Their long, slender microvilli extend toward the photoreceptors and surround the outer segments. Other apical cell processes have a cup shape to envelop an outer segment. The pigment epithelial cells contain lysosomes to digest the shed fragments. The mitochondria are plentiful, as these cells are obligately aerobic. The melanosomes are considerably larger than their counterparts in the uveal stroma and are of two types, spherical and elongated. The pigment epithelial cell nuclei are round and are found toward the base of the cell. The basal cytoplasmic membrane shows considerable infolding.

There are no tight junctions between the pigment epithelium and the photoreceptors. Instead, other forces keep the two layers apposed in the living eye. The interphotoreceptor matrix proteins provide a powerful adhesive force. However, the main attractive force is the vacuum created by the pigment epithelium through active transport. Several ion transport systems are present in the retinal pigment epithelium, and these differ for the apical surface and the basal surface. The net effect is that ions are transported away from the retinal side of the cell toward the choroidal side, and water follows the ions away from the subsensory retinal potential space.

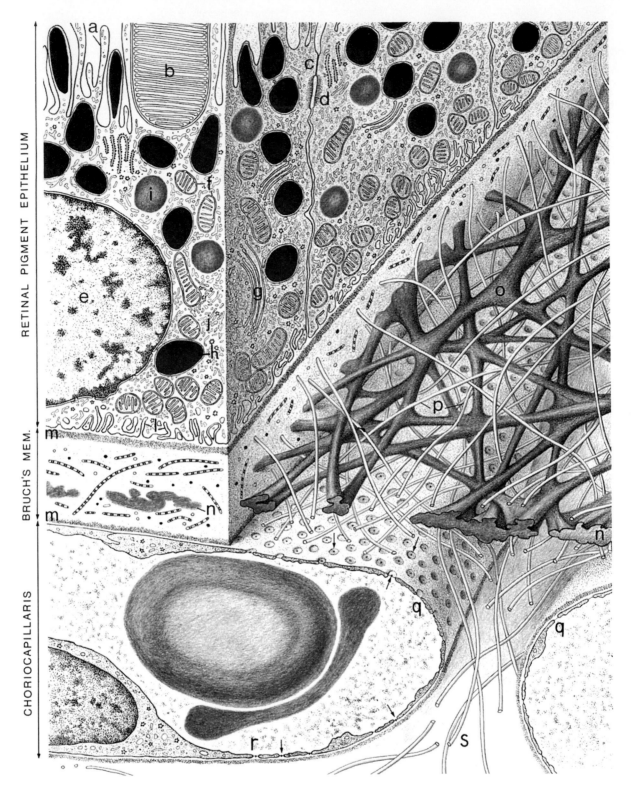

Fig. 9-1   Three-dimensional drawing of the inner choroid and retinal pigment epithelium. The villi of the pigment epithelium *(a)* extend internally to enclose the outer segments of the rods and cones *(b)*. The intercellular junctions are characterized by a zonula occludens *(c)* and a desmosome *(d);* otherwise, the cell relations are of the usual type. The cytoplasm of the pigment cells contains a nucleus *(e)*, mitochondria *(f)*, a Golgi apparatus *(g)*, pigment granules *(h)*, and phagosomes *(i)*, and it is characterized by a large amount of smooth-surfaced endoplasmic reticulum *(j)*. The external cell membrane shows complex infoldings *(l)* and a basement membrane *(m)*. Bruch's membrane shows an apparently interrupted elastic zone (n) in meridional section, but the elastica is layered and continuous in flat section *(o)*. Collagen fibrins *(p)* that form the inner and outer collagenous zones have a random orientation around the elastic zone. The choriocapillaris *(q)* shows a fenestrated endothelium internally, laterally, and, to a lesser extent, externally *(r)*. The intercapillary zone shows considerable collagen *(s)*. The lumen of the capillary contains two red blood cells. (From Hogan MA, Alvarado J, Weddell J: *Histology of the eye,* Philadelphia, 1971, WB Saunders.)

Each pigment epithelial cell is bound to its neighbor by a tight junction. These junctions encircle the cells toward their apices and serve to prevent extracellular molecules from entering the subsensory retinal space. This complex of junctions, the zonulae adherentes and zonulae occludentes, are referred to collectively as the outer blood-retinal barrier, analogous to the blood-brain barrier. Small molecules (such as fluorescein) can diffuse inward from the choriocapillaris, through Bruch's membrane and between adjacent retinal pigment epithelial cells, but ordinarily cannot gain access to the subretinal space.

BRUCH'S MEMBRANE

Between the base of the retinal pigment epithelium and the choriocapillaris is Bruch's membrane, a five-layer structure. From outward to inward, it consists of the basement membrane of the choriocapillaris, a layer of collagen, an elastic layer, another layer of collagen, and finally the basement membrane of the retinal pigment epithelium.

SENSORY RETINA: THREE BANDS OF NUCLEI

In contrast to the outer neuroectodermal layer, which normally remains a monolayer, the inner neuroectodermal layer proliferates early in embryonic life to form what is obviously a complex multilayered structure (Fig. 9-2). Clinically, the sensory retina lines most of the inner aspect of the eye, from the optic nerve head posteriorly to the ora serrata anteriorly. The peripheral margin of the sensory retina, the ora serrata, is scalloped, especially nasally. The ora serrata approximately overlies the insertions of the rectus muscles.

By light microscopy, three bands of nuclei are apparent, separated by bands of nonnuclear material. This ordered structure is reminiscent of, although certainly not identical with, cerebral and cerebellar cortex, underscoring the retina's identity as a central nervous system structure.

It is easiest to understand the retinal layers in terms of their function. The outermost layer of nuclei is called the outer nuclear layer. These are the nuclei of the photoreceptors. External to the nuclei are the inner segments and then the outer segments of these specialized cells.

Photoreceptors

As befits their function, rod and cone cells are unique, elongated cells (Fig. 9-3). There are approximately 130 million rods and about 7 million cones in each human retina. Rods are sensitive to dim light; theoretical calculation indicates that a rod cell can perceive a single photon of light. Thus they are primarily responsible for peripheral vision and vision under scotopic conditions. The outer segments of rods consist of a series of stacked unit-membrane discs, about 1000 per rod outer segment. These discs are separate from the plasma membrane in the rod, but they remain continuous with it in the cone.

The outer segments of the rods and cones contain the light-sensitive molecules. The rods contain rhodopsin, a complex of opsin, a glycoprotein, coupled with 11-*cis*-retinaldehyde, the chromophore. Rhodopsin is a membrane-bound protein. It weaves in and out of the cell membrane seven times, so that portions of the molecule are intracytoplasmic, portions are within the lumen of the stacked disc, and portions are within the membrane itself. Mutations have been identified in several locations along the rhodopsin molecule that lead to various types of retinitis pigmentosa.

When a photon of light strikes the rhodopsin molecule, called "bleaching," an isomerization ensues, so

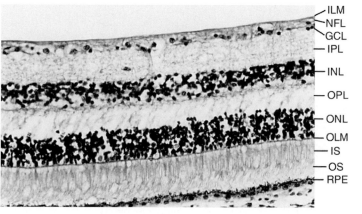

Fig. 9-2 Layers of the retina. The retinal pigment epithelium *(RPE)* is adjacent to the photoreceptor outer segments *(OS)*, which in turn connect to the inner segments *(IS)*. The Müller cells and photoreceptors have tight junctions between them, seen just below the outer nuclear layer. Because the retinal structure is so orderly, these junctions form a straight line, the outer limiting membrane (OLM). However, it is not a true membrane. The photoreceptor nuclei are the nuclei of the outer nuclear layer *(ONL)*. Synapses take place between the photoreceptors and the cells of the inner nuclear layer *(INL)* in the outer plexiform layer *(OPL)*. The cells of the inner nuclear layer in turn synapse with the ganglion cells *(GCL)* in the inner plexiform layer *(IPL)*. The axons of the ganglion cells together comprise the nerve fiber layer *(NFL)*. Innermost, and next to the vitreous, is the internal limiting membrane *(ILM)*. Hematoxylin and eosin, ×200. (See color plate.)

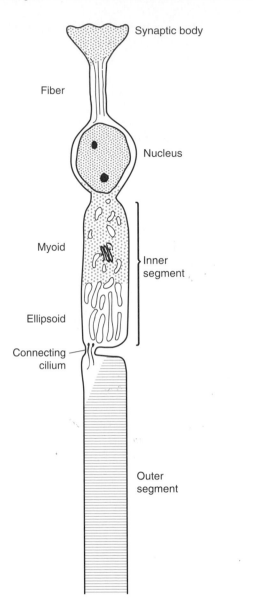

Fig. 9-3   Diagram illustrating the basic organization of a vertebrate visual cell. (From Young RW: Visual cells and the concept of renewal, *Invest Ophthalmol Vis Sci* 15:700-725, 1976.)

that 11-*cis*-retinaldehyde is transformed to 11-*trans*-retinaldehyde. Because the isomerization changes the shape of the molecule, the all-*trans*-retinaldehyde is now unable to bind properly to the opsin (Fig. 9-4). A series of light-independent (so-called "dark") reactions ensues within the photoreceptor and the enveloping pigment epithelial cell, which ultimately leads to the regeneration of the original rhodopsin molecule. Meanwhile, a neural impulse has been generated.

The cones are responsible for fine visual discrimination and for color vision. The cone outer segments are shorter and tapered, giving them their name. They also consist of stacked discs containing visual pigments, but the discs are continuous with the cell membrane rather than separate from it, as in the rods. There are three types, formerly referred to as red, green, and blue cones, but they now are characterized as long, medium, and short (L, M, and S), respectively, based on the relative wavelength in the visible spectrum to which they are sensitive. The L and M photopigments are actually very similar structurally, and both are coded on the X chromosome. The S photopigment is coded on chromosome 7; defects of this class are much more rare than abnormalities of either the L or M photoreceptors.

The relative populations and spatial distributions of these three classes of cones seem to be random and variable, as measured in the living eye. However, although cones are found throughout the retina, they are most concentrated in the macula, especially the fovea (Fig. 9-5). At the center of the fovea, they are so crowded that the outer segments are elongated and appear morphologically rodlike.

The stacked discs of the rod are constantly shed. The shed discs are taken up and digested by the retinal pigment epithelium. Cone discs are shed also, but the mechanism is less well understood. New discs are synthesized by the organelles of the inner segment.

The inner segment of both the rod and the cone is connected to the outer segment by a nonmotile cilium. Within the inner segments are abundant mitochondria,

Fig. 9-4   The change in configuration of the rhodopsin molecule as it is activated by absorption of a photon of light. (From Newell FW: *Ophthalmology, principles and concepts,* ed 7, St Louis, 1992, Mosby.)

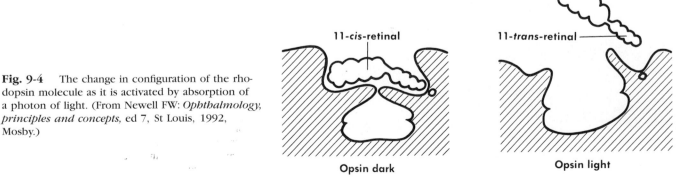

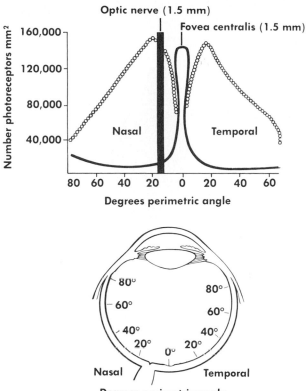

Fig. 9-5   The density of retinal rods and cones as a function of retinal location. The cones are concentrated in the fovea centralis (0°). The rod density peaks at about 20° from the fovea centralis and gradually diminishes to the retinal periphery. There are no rods at the fovea centralis. (From Newell FW: *Ophthalmology, principles and concepts,* ed 7, St Louis, 1992, Mosby.)

indicating their active aerobic metabolic status. Other organelles are also present.

The rods and cones both have receptor terminals on their inner aspects, sites where they synapse with the next layer of cells (Fig. 9-6). In rods, these terminals are small and are called pedicles. In cones they are larger and are called spherules.

Inner Nuclear Layer

The next layer of nuclei is the inner nuclear layer. Within this layer are a number of different types of neurons: bipolar cells, amacrine cells, horizontal cells, and interplexiform cells. Between these two layers, the inner and outer retinal layers, is a layer without nuclei, the outer plexiform layer. (Some have called this the outer synaptic layer, a more functionally descriptive term.) Synapses between the photoreceptors and these other neurons take place in the outer plexiform layer. The interactions of these different types of cells are complex and include synapses with other cells of the inner nuclear

layer, as well as with the photoreceptors and ganglion cell layers.

Ganglion Cell Layer

The cells of the inner nuclear layer in turn synapse in the inner plexiform layer with the cells of the ganglion cell layer. This is the innermost of the three nuclear layers. Away from the anatomic macula, this layer is essentially one cell layer thick. The ganglion cells are larger and have paler nuclei than the cells of the other two layers. Each ganglion cell has a single axon. Collectively, most of these axons form the nerve fiber layer, which proceeds centripetally to the optic nerve to exit the eye. However, there are about 2 million ganglion cells in the retina, but only about 1.25 million axons in the optic nerve. The other axons remain within the retina.

The nasal fibers proceed more or less directly to the optic nerve, but the fibers temporal to the nerve sweep around the macula (Fig. 9-7). The fibers from the fovea itself are numerous, so that about 65% of all the axons of the retina are located in the papillomacular bundle.

Inward from the nerve fiber layer is the internal limiting membrane. This is a basement membrane secreted by the Müller cells, a type of glial cell. Müller cells are also derived from neuroectoderm and in fact are the only cells of the sensory retina that maintain this basal attachment (Fig. 9-8). They elongate to span virtually the entire thickness of the retina. At their outermost extent, the Müller cells form tight junctions with the adjacent photoreceptors. Because of the ordered structure of the retina, these junctions can appear as a line just external to the outer nuclear layer. This line is sometimes referred to as the outer limiting membrane, but it is not a membrane, as demonstrated by electron microscopy. A similar but less conspicuous series of junctions, the middle limiting membrane, is sometimes visible just external to the inner nuclear layer.

The nuclei of the Müller cells reside in the inner nuclear layer. Müller cells are believed to have support and nutritive functions, analogous to the astrocytes of the central nervous system.

MACULA

The macula is that specialized area of the retina primarily involved in photopic vision; that is, color vision and central vision.

The anatomist and the clinician use the term "macula" differently, mostly because the clinical landmarks have no exact histologic counterparts and vice versa (Fig. 9-9). The anatomic macula is about 5.5 mm in diameter and is defined as that area of the retina where the ganglion cell layer is greater than a single nucleus thick. This

Text continued on p. 71

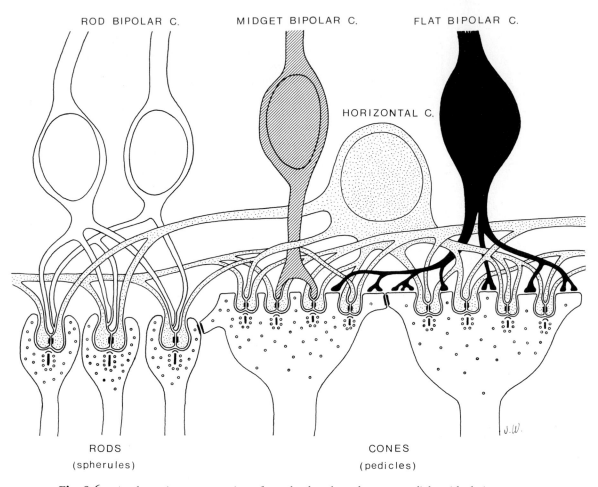

Fig. 9-6   A schematic representation of a rod spherule and a cone pedicle with their synapses. Rod and cone bipolar cells show extensive contacts. The horizontal cells also make synapses with both the rods and the cones. Interconnections are also shown between rod spherules and cone pedicles. (Modified from Dowling JE, Boycott BB: Organization of the primate retina: electron microscopy, *Proc Roy Soc London B Biol Sci* 166:80-111, 1966.)

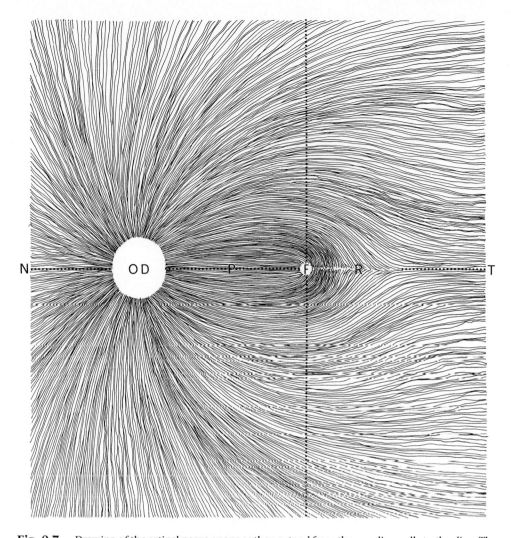

Fig. 9-7   Drawing of the retinal nerve axons as they extend from the ganglion cells to the disc. The superior, inferior, and nasal axons are fairly straight. The course of the temporal axons is curved and becomes increasingly more curved in the macular region. The axons arising from the nasal macula extend directly toward the optic disc *(OD)* as the papillomacular bundle *(P)*. Temporal to the fovea *(F)* is the horizontal raphe *(R)*. In the region of the raphe the courses of the axons are of three types—vertical, oblique, and triangular. The vertical axons are more numerous. The dotted lines delineate the nasal, temporal, superior, and inferior hemiretina. *N,* Nasal; *T,* temporal. (From Hogan MA, Alvarado J, Weddell J: *Histology of the eye,* Philadelphia, 1971, WB Saunders.)

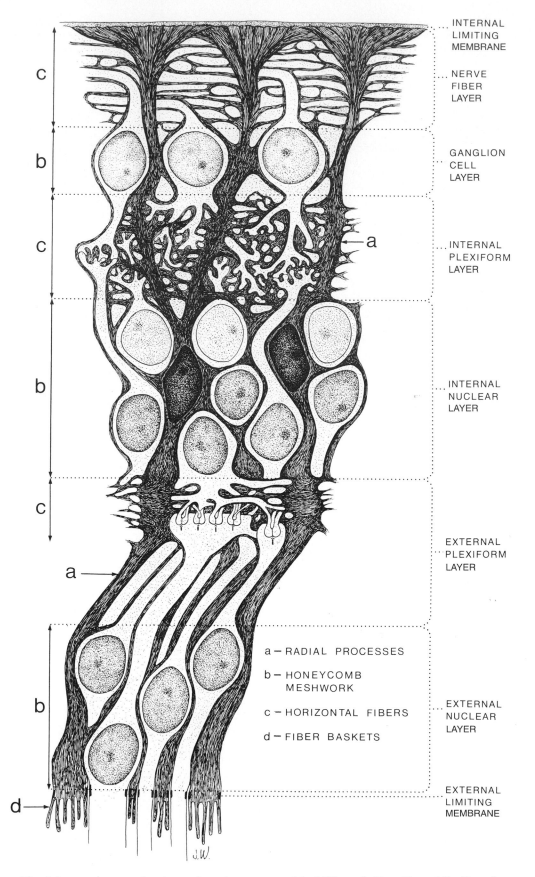

Fig. 9-8   A schematic drawing to show the structure of the Müller cell. (From Hogan MA, Alvarado J, Weddell J: *Histology of the eye,* Philadelphia, 1971, WB Saunders.)

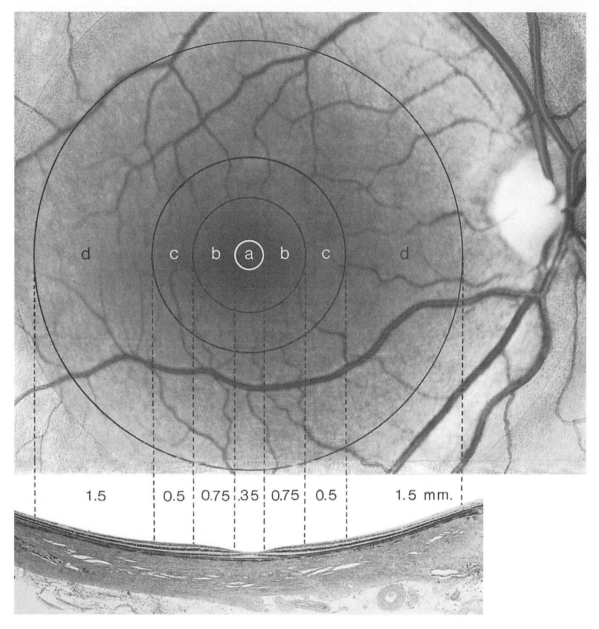

1.5 | 0.5 | 0.75 |.35| 0.75 | 0.5 | 1.5 mm.

Fig. 9-9   This fundus photograph is matched with a meridional light micrograph of the macular region. The fundus photograph shows the foveola *(a)*, fovea *(b)*, parafoveal area *(c)*, and perifoveal region *(d)*. (From Hogan MA, Alvarado J, Weddell J: *Histology of the eye,* Philadelphia, 1971, WB Saunders.)

corresponds very approximately to the clinician's posterior pole. What is clinically referred to as the macula corresponds to the anatomic fovea, the central depressed area that is about 1.5 mm in diameter, or about the size of the optic nerve head. In younger persons, it is often outlined by an oval light reflex, with the horizontal diameter slightly larger. The anatomic foveola, approximately the size of the clinical fovea, is the central floor of the pit and is about 350 μ in diameter. (For com-

parison, the foveal avascular zone is about 500 μ in diameter.) In young people, there is often a tiny bright spot of light, a virtual image created by the parabolic reflection from the pit. In this area, the only photoreceptors are cones, and because of the tight packing, they are elongated and slender, morphologically resembling rods.

Microscopically, the foveola consists only of photoreceptors and some Müller cells (Fig. 9-10). The other layers, from the outer plexiform layer inward, are pushed to

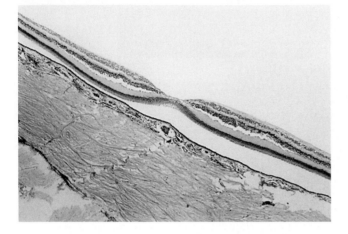

Fig. 9-10   Low-power view of the fovea and foveola. Even at this power, we can see that the inner two nuclear layers are discontinuous at the foveal pit. Hematoxylin and eosin, ×20. (See color plate.)

the side. This modification, along with the avascularity, presumably ensures the least possible interference with incident light, allowing optimal vision.

The macula has a yellow color, imparted mainly by a carotenoid called lutein. Its function is probably to act as a filter to minimize light scatter. It is dissolved out of routine histologic preparations but can be observed and characterized through specialized techniques. The xanthophyll pigment is located primarily in the outer and inner plexiform layers.

Periphery

Anatomically, all the retina except for the macula is defined as retinal periphery. However, clinically the periphery tends to be defined as the area anterior to the equator.

The ora serrata forms the junction between ciliary epithelium and the retina. It has a scalloped configuration, especially superonasally where the teeth, or dentate processes, are longer and the bays are deeper. Microscopically, the transition between sensory retina and ciliary epithelium is abrupt.

There are congenital variant forms of the teeth and bays. Meridional folds are meridionally oriented tented-up areas; sometimes such a fold extends far enough anteriorly that it meets with a ciliary process. These are called meridional complexes. Oral bays can be unusually deep, bounded on either side by large dentate processes, called giant teeth. If the bay is closed by these two teeth, there is an "island" of pars plana with retina both anterior and posterior to this island. This is called an enclosed oral bay.

Blood Supply

The vascular supply to the retina comes from two sources. The outer retina is supplied by diffusion from the choroid, whereas the inner retina is supplied by the retinal vascular system. These systems do not normally contact each other, and there is very little overlap between them. We know this because natural "experiments" show that the retinal circulation supplies the inner retina outward to include a portion of the inner nuclear layer; these inner layers are lost with a complete retinal arterial occlusion (central or branch). In contrast, vascular occlusion in peripheral choroid results in cobblestone or paving stone degeneration; microscopically these lesions show loss of retinal pigment epithelium and outer retinal layers.

The ophthalmic artery is the first branch of the internal carotid artery. In turn, the retinal artery is the first branch of the ophthalmic artery. The central retinal artery enters the optic nerve from approximately 10 mm posterior to the eye and travels within the nerve until it enters the eye. Almost immediately, the vessel divides to form four branches. The nasal branches extend superiorly and inferiorly, and the two temporal branches run superior and inferior to the macula in an arcuate configuration. As the vessels proceed peripherally, they branch further. The returning venules more or less follow the arterioles. The precise pattern of the vessels is unique to each eye.

The retinal vessels share morphologic characteristics with those of the brain. The arteries are end vessels, normally without anastomoses; thus closure of one such vessel causes infarction of its territory. Another similarity is the lack of capillary fenestrations. Retinal capillaries, like those of the brain, do not leak small molecules such as fluorescein. (In contrast, capillaries elsewhere in the eye and the body freely leak fluorescein.) The retinal capillaries form the second blood-retinal barrier.

Cilioretinal arteries, if present, enter the retina from the choroid at the margin of the optic nerve. Thus they are not part of the retinal circulation, but rather fill as the choroidal vasculature does, a second or so before the retinal vessels originating from the central retinal artery. Not all individuals have a cilioretinal artery, and the area of retina supplied by such a vessel ranges from trivial to the entire posterior pole. Even though these vessels do not originate from the central retinal artery, they have permeability characteristics similar to those of the rest of the retinal circulation.

Vitreous

The vitreous occupies much of the eye and acts as structural support to the retina. It is a gel of cross-linked

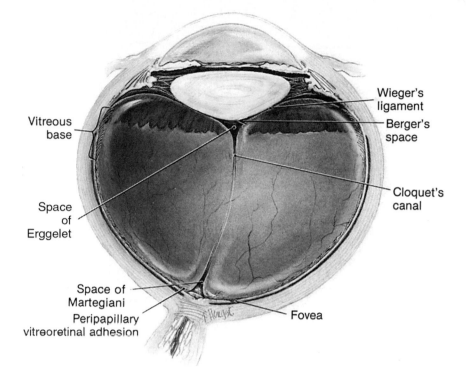

Fig. 9-11   Primary and secondary vitreous relations and attachments to surrounding tissues in childhood and early adult life. Remnants of primary vitreous constitute Cloquet's canal extending from the posterior lens surface (Wieger's ligament) to the peripheral margin of optic nerve. Secondary vitreous adheres to adjacent tissues in region of the vitreous base and optic nerve with less firm attachment surrounding the fovea. Collagen fibers in cortical vitreous gel are parallel to retina posteriorly and perpendicular to the retina at the vitreous base. (From Michels RG: *Vitreous surgery*, St Louis, 1981, Mosby. Copyright © Johns Hopkins University.)

collagen fibers along with hyaluronic acid, apparently secreted during embryonic life by the inner retinal cells. Fibers extend through the internal limiting membrane to attach to the Müller cell footplates. Occasional hyalocytes are present; they may have synthetic and phagocytic functions. They become less numerous with age.

At the slit lamp, we see a central canal making a gentle S shape from over the optic nerve head to the posterior aspect of the lens. This is Cloquet's canal, the remnant of the primary vitreous (Fig. 9-11). It widens both anteriorly and posteriorly to form the spaces of Berger and of Martegiani, respectively.

The attachment between the vitreous and surrounding tissues is strongest at the vitreous base, a band 2 to 6 mm in width straddling the peripheral retina and posterior pars plana (Fig. 9-12). This bond remains strong throughout life. Other, weaker attachments exist surrounding the optic nerve, overlying the macula, and running along the major vessels of the retina.

Electron microscopy of fresh vitreous shows it to be a structureless gel. Collagen fibrils 10 to 25 nm in diameter with 22 nm periodicity are most dense near the retina, especially anteriorly and least so centrally.

The vitreous is about 99% water; most of the solid material is collagen, primarily types II, XI, and IX. The hyaluronic acid acts to trap and maintain the high water content. This is a dynamic process, as the half-time of water turnover is about 10 to 15 minutes.

OPTIC NERVE

The approximately 1.25 million axons of the nerve fiber layer come together to exit the eye as the optic nerve. As befits a central nervous system structure, the accompanying glial cells include astrocytes.

The optic nerve head is slightly larger vertically than horizontally. Centrally there is a round or slightly oval depression, the optic cup. Normally, the diameter of the cup is no larger than one-third of the diameter of the optic disc.

The blood supply of the optic nerve head has been a matter of controversy in terms of the relative contribu-

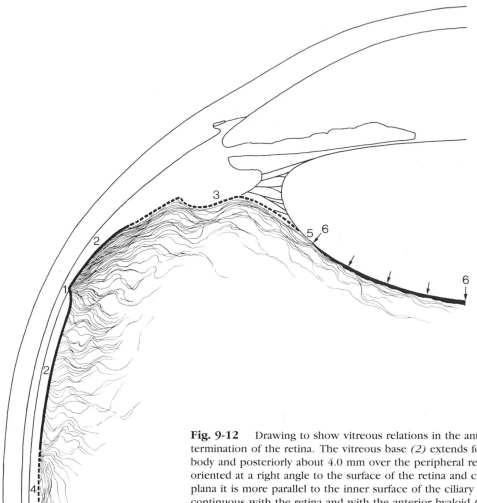

Fig. 9-12 Drawing to show vitreous relations in the anterior eye. The ora serrata *(1)* is the termination of the retina. The vitreous base *(2)* extends forward about 2.0 mm over the ciliary body and posteriorly about 4.0 mm over the peripheral retina. The collagen in this region is oriented at a right angle to the surface of the retina and ciliary body, but anteriorly over the pars plana it is more parallel to the inner surface of the ciliary body. The posterior hyaloid *(4)* is continuous with the retina and with the anterior hyaloid *(3)* with the zonules and lens. The ligamentum pectinatum is at *5* and the space of Berger is at *6*. (From Hogan MA, Alvarado J, Weddell J: *Histology of the eye,* Philadelphia, 1971, WB Saunders.)

tions of the different components. It appears, however, that this 0.7-mm segment is perfused primarily by branches of the posterior ciliary arteries and also by retinal arterioles.

The optic nerve, as it exits the eye, must traverse the sclera (Fig. 9-13). In this area, the sclera is continuous with a porous structure, the lamina cribrosa (see Fig. 4-9). The pores are larger superiorly and inferiorly than they are nasally and temporally.

Just past the lamina cribrosa, the optic nerve becomes myelinated. It therefore also becomes much larger in size, 3 mm in diameter.

The retrobulbar optic nerve can be divided into regions: the intraocular, the intraorbital, the intracanalicular, and the intracranial portions. The intraocular portion is only 0.7 mm; this length corresponds to the thickness of the sclera and retina.

The intraorbital portion is 33 mm. This is longer than the distance from the orbital apex to the posterior sur-

face of the eyeball. There must be some slack for ocular movement, so in its primary position the optic nerve assumes a somewhat S shape. The central retinal artery and vein enter the nerve approximately 10 mm behind the globe (Fig. 9-14).

The optic nerve continues posteriorly within the muscle cone to the orbital canal. Here it is tethered by the dura, which fuses with the periosteum of the canal. Thus while the nerve moves freely within the orbit, it is fixed posterior to the orbit.

The intracanalicular portion of the optic nerve is 6 mm in length, and the intracranial portion, from its entry to the chiasm, is 10 mm.

Meninges

At the optic canal at the apex of the orbit, the dural sheath of the optic nerve becomes continuous with the periosteum. This is also true on the intracranial side

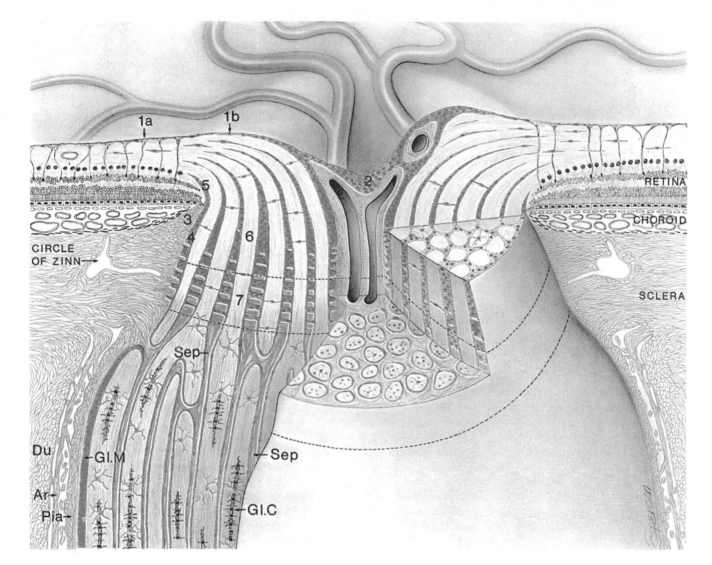

Fig. 9-13   Three-dimensional color drawing of the intraocular and part of the orbital optic nerve. Where the retina terminates at the optic disc edge, the Müller cells *(1a)* are in continuity with the astrocytes, forming the *internal limiting membrane of Elschnig (1b)*. In some specimens Elschnig's membrane is thickened in the central portion of the disc to form the *central meniscus of Kuhnt (2)*. At the posterior termination of the choroids on the temporal side, the border tissue of Elschnig *(3)* lies between the astrocytes surrounding the optic nerve canal *(4)* and the stroma of the choroids. On the nasal side, the choroidal stroma is directly adjacent to the astrocytes surrounding the nerve. This collection of astrocytes *(4)* surrounding the canal is known as the border *tissue of Jacoby*. This is continuous with a similar glial lining called the intermediary tissue of Kuhnt *(5)* at the termination of the retina. The nerve fibers of the retina are segregated into approximately 1000 bundles or fascicles by astrocytes *(6)*. Upon reaching the lamina cribrosa (upper dotted line), the nerve fascicles *(7)* and their surrounding astrocytes are separated from each other by connective tissue (drawn in blue). This connective tissue is the cribriform plate, which is an extension of scleral collagen and elastic fibers through the nerve. The external choroid also sends some connective tissue to the anterior part of the lamina. At the external part of the lamina cribrosa (lower dotted line), the nerve fibers become myelinated and columns of oligodendrocytes (black and white cells) and a few astrocytes (red-colored cells) are present within the nerve fascicles. The astrocytes surrounding the fascicles form a thinner layer here than in the laminar and prelaminar portion. The bundles continue to be separated by connective tissue all the way to the chiasm *(Sep)*. This connective tissue is derived from the pia mater and is known as the septal tissue. A mantle of astrocytes *(Gl.M)*, continuous anteriorly with the border tissue of Jacoby, surrounds the nerve along its orbital course. The dura *(Du)*, arachnoid *(Ar)*, and pia mater *(Pia)* are shown. The central retinal vessels are surrounded by a perivascular connective tissue throughout its course in the nerve. This connective tissue blends with the connective tissue of the cribriform plate in the lamina cribrosa; it is called the central supporting connective tissue strand here. (From Anderson D, Hoyt W: Ultrastructure of intraorbital portion of human and monkey optic nerve, *Arch Ophthalmol* 82:506-530, 1969.) (See color plate.)

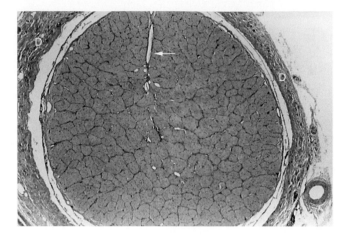

Fig. 9-14 The optic nerve in cross section with the surrounding dural sheath *(D).* The bundles of axons are evident. The central retinal vessels have entered the nerve *(arrow).* Hematoxylin and eosin, ×20. (See color plate.)

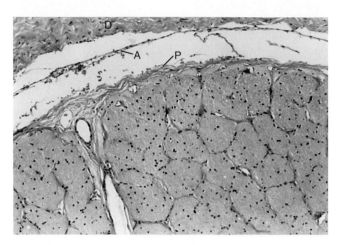

Fig. 9-15 Higher-power view of the optic nerve, showing the dura *(D),* arachnoid *(A),* and pia *(P).* The pial septa surround bundles of axons. The nuclei are astrocytes. Hematoxylin and eosin, ×20. (See color plate.)

MAJOR POINTS

The retina is an extension of the brain. Light stimuli are received by the photoreceptors and partially processed within the retina before being sent to the brain via the optic nerve.

All stimuli to the retina, including heat, cold, and pressure, are interpreted by the brain as light.

The sensory retina consists of three bands of nuclei. The outermost band includes the nuclei of the photoreceptors. The middle band (inner nuclear layer) includes nuclei of amacrine, bipolar, interplexiform, and horizontal cells. The innermost band includes the ganglion cell nuclei.

Synapses between these layers of nuclei take place in the outer and inner plexiform layers.

The nerve fiber layer consists of the axons of the ganglion cells, most of which go centripetally to exit the eye as the optic nerve.

There are two blood-retinal barriers. The outer barrier, at the apex of the retinal pigment epithelial cells, is formed by the tight junctions binding each cell to its neighbors. The inner barrier is the nonfenestrated endothelial cells of the retinal capillaries.

The retinal pigment epithelium participates in regeneration of rhodopsin, the visual pigment. It also phagocytizes the shed outer segments of the rods and cones.

The sensory retina remains attached to the pigment epithelium primarily through a vacuum created by its ion transport systems. Disruption of these can lead to retinal detachment.

The internal limiting membrane is the basement membrane of the Müller cells, support cells that run almost the entire thickness of the retina. The so-called external and middle limiting "membranes" are a series of tight junctions between Müller cells and the photoreceptors and cells of the inner nuclear layer, respectively.

The anatomic macula is about 5.5 mm in diameter, approximately the area within the superior and inferior temporal vascular arcades. In the anatomic macula, the ganglion cell layer is more than a single cell nucleus thick.

The floor of the fovea contains only cones, although they are so compressed that they are morphologically rodlike. All other layers are pushed aside. A few Müller cells are also present in the fovea.

The macula contains a xanthophyll pigment, primarily in the outer and inner plexiform layers.

The retina becomes continuous with the ciliary epithelium at the ora serrata. Its scallops are most pronounced superonasally.

The choroidal vasculature supplies the retinal pigment epithelium and outer aspect of the retina via diffusion.

The inner aspect of the retina is supplied by the retinal vasculature. The boundary between the two blood supplies is in the midst of the inner nuclear layer.

The vitreous is a gel of cross-linked collagen with hyaluronic acid. The collagen is most dense peripherally, near the retina.

The strongest attachment between the vitreous and retina is at the vitreous base at the retinal periphery. Strong attachments also occur around the optic nerve head, over the macula, and along major vessels.

The optic nerve consists of ganglion cell axons, which become myelinated past the lamina cribrosa.

The optic nerve is surrounded by the meninges, dura, arachnoid, and pia. The fibrovascular pial septa surround columns of axons, and the pial vasculature is the primary blood supply.

of the canal and means that the subdural space of the optic nerve is not continuous with the intracranial subdural space. (However, the subarachnoid space is continuous.) This firm attachment of the dura to the orbital periosteum serves to act as an anchor for the optic nerve.

The pia, unlike the dura and arachnoid, not only surrounds the optic nerve as a whole but also penetrates its substance to surround the axon bundles (Fig. 9-15). Thus this meninx cannot be stripped from the optic nerve because it is an integral part of the optic nerve structure. The pial septa consist of fibrovascular tissue and serve a structural and nutritive function. Posterior to the globe, the primary blood supply to the nerve is the pial vasculature.

SUGGESTED READINGS

Asrani S, Zou S, d'Anna S, et al: Noninvasive mapping of the normal retinal thickness at the posterior pole, *Ophthalmology* 106:269-273, 1999.

Bok D: Retinal photoreceptor-pigment epithelium interactions, *Invest Ophthalmol Vis Sci* 26:1659, 1985.

Cunha-Vaz J: The blood-ocular barriers, *Surv Ophthalmol* 23: 279-296, 1979.

Dowling JE: *The retina: an approachable part of the brain,* Cambridge, Mass, 1987, Belknap Press of Harvard University.

Duvall J: Structure, function, and pathologic responses of pigment epithelium: a review, *Semin Ophthalmol* 2:130-140, 1987.

Gass JDM: Muller cell cone, an overlooked part of the anatomy of the fovea centralis, *Arch Ophthalmol* 117:821-823, 1999.

Gentile RC, Berinstein DM, Leibmann J, et al: High-resolution ultrasound biomicroscopy of the pars plana and peripheral retina, *Ophthalmology* 105:478-484, 1998.

Hageman GS, Marmor MF, Yao XY, Johnson LV: The interphotoreceptor matrix mediates primate retinal adhesion, *Arch Ophthalmol* 113:655-660,1995.

Justice J Jr, Lehmann RP: Cilioretinal arteries: a study based on review of stereo fundus photographs and fluorescein angiographic findings, *Arch Ophthalmol* 94:1355-1358, 1976.

Neitz M, Neitz J: Molecular genetics of color vision and color vision defects, *Arch Ophthalmol* 118:691-700, 2000.

Roorda A, Williams DR: The arrangement of the three cone classes in the living human eye, *Nature* 397:520-522, 1999.

Sebag J: Age-related differences in the human vitreoretinal interface, *Arch Ophthalmol* 109:966-971, 1991.

Orbit and Adnexa: Protection and Support

BONY ORBIT

EXTRAOCULAR MUSCLES

FASCIA

NERVES AND CILIARY GANGLION

BLOOD SUPPLY

The eye must be exposed to the world to function, yet as a consequence it is vulnerable to external trauma. How can it be protected? The bony orbit acts as a partially surrounding shield, and the fat that fills much of the orbit forms a cushion and shock absorber. The result is a remarkably efficient protective apparatus.

BONY ORBIT

The bony orbit is shaped approximately like a four-sided pyramid that bulges near its base (Fig. 10-1). Anteriorly, the orbital rim is thick and strong, especially superiorly; this acts to protect the eye. Although of course the bones form a continuum, it can be helpful to think of them as forming four discrete walls (Box 10-1).

The superior wall of the orbit serves to separate the eye from the frontal lobe of the brain. The bones of this side are relatively thin posterior to the rim. The frontal bone comprises most of the superior wall, while the lesser wing of the sphenoid forms the optic canal and separates it from the superior orbital fissure. Within the frontal bone are the frontal sinuses; these vary considerably in size, even between the two sides in the same individual.

The lateral wall is comprised of two bones. Anteriorly, the zygomatic bone forms the thick and strong lateral rim and extends back to join the greater wing of the sphenoid posteriorly.

The inferior wall is comprised of three bones. Anteriorly, the maxillary bone forms the orbital rim, and, as it runs posteriorly, it separates the orbit from the max-

illary sinus. The orbital floor is the most vulnerable to traumatic fracture, because it is quite thin posterior to the rim. A portion of the zygomatic bone contributes to the inferior wall, as does a small portion of the palatine bone posteriorly.

The medial wall separates the eye from the ethmoid and sphenoid sinuses. This wall is comprised of four bones, the maxilla, and the lacrimal, ethmoid, and sphenoid bones. The maxilla and the lacrimal bone serve to support the lacrimal sac and duct. Although the ethmoid bone is actually the thinnest of all the orbital bones, the structure of the sinus and the bony walls between resembles corrugated cardboard, giving the medial wall relatively greater strength than would be expected on the basis of thickness alone.

At the apex are two large openings, the optic canal and the orbital fissure (Fig. 10-2). Both are formed by the sphenoid bone. The optic nerve is the only structure exiting through the optic canal. The orbital fissure is a boomerang-shaped opening just lateral to the optic canal. Nothing enters through the inferior portion. However, the superior orbital fissure is a conduit for a number of nerves and vessels (Box 10-2).

EXTRAOCULAR MUSCLES

The extraocular muscles, as their name implies, control the movements of the two eyes in space. There are 12 in all, 6 per eye. Of these, 4 are rectus muscles and 2 are oblique muscles.

Except for the inferior oblique muscle, the extraocular muscles, along with the levator muscle, originate at the orbital apex at the annulus of Zinn. These muscle origins form a fibrous ring that surrounds the optic nerve. Within the ring are the nerves that innervate the muscles, the superior and inferior branches of cranial nerve III, and cranial nerve VI. These motor nerves run

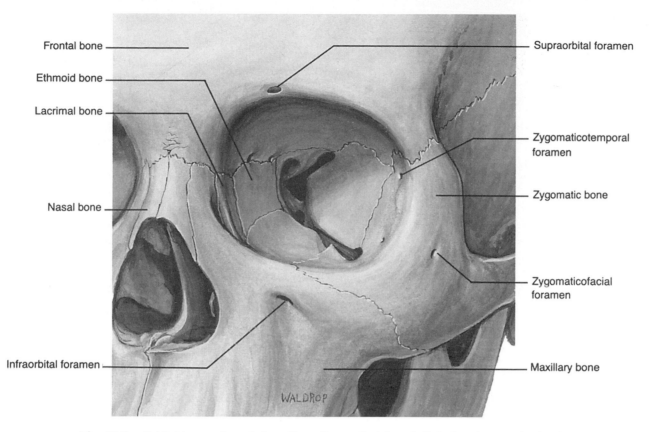

Frontal bone

Ethmoid bone

Lacrimal bone

Nasal bone

Infraorbital foramen

Supraorbital foramen

Zygomaticotemporal foramen

Zygomatic bone

Zygomaticofacial foramen

Maxillary bone

WALDROP

Fig. 10-1   Orbital bones, frontal view. (From Dutton JJ. *Atlas of clinical and surgical orbital anatomy*, Philadelphia, 1994, WB Saunders.) (See color plate.)

Box 10-1 **Bones of the Orbit**	
SUPERIOR WALL	**INFERIOR WALL**
Frontal bone	Maxilla
Lesser wing of sphenoid	Zygoma
	Palatine
LATERAL WALL	**MEDIAL WALL**
Zygoma	Maxilla
Greater wing of sphenoid	Lacrimal
	Ethmoid
	Sphenoid

along the inner aspects of the muscle bellies. The superior branch of cranial nerve III innervates the levator and the superior rectus muscles, the inferior branch innervates the inferior and medial rectus and inferior oblique muscles, and cranial nerve VI innervates the lateral rectus muscle (Box 10-3).

The trochlear nerve, cranial nerve IV, however, enters the orbit through the superior orbital fissure but superior to the muscle annulus. It crosses external to the levator,

running medially until it contacts the medial aspect of the superior oblique muscle.

The muscles diverge from each other as they advance anteriorly, forming the muscle cone. The four rectus muscles attach to the eye anterior to the equator. As we realize intuitively, the medial rectus muscle pulls the eye medially and the lateral rectus pulls it laterally.

However, the vertical rectus muscles do not move the eye in quite so straightforward a manner. The central axis of the orbit is not parallel to the visual axis. Instead, the medial orbital walls are essentially parallel to each other, but the lateral walls form a right angle (see Fig. 3-2). Thus the axis of the eye forms a 22.5° angle with the axis of the orbit. In turn, this implies that the superior and inferior rectus muscles each have a torsional effect as well as their primary effect of raising and lowering the eye, respectively.

The inferior oblique muscle is the only muscle that does not arise in the orbital apex. It originates medially in the orbit and sweeps under the inferior rectus muscle to attach to the globe temporal to the optic nerve.

The superior oblique muscle swings anteromedial to enter the trochlea. This is a fibrocartilaginous structure just posterior to the orbital rim superomedially. The tendon of the superior oblique muscle then courses poste-

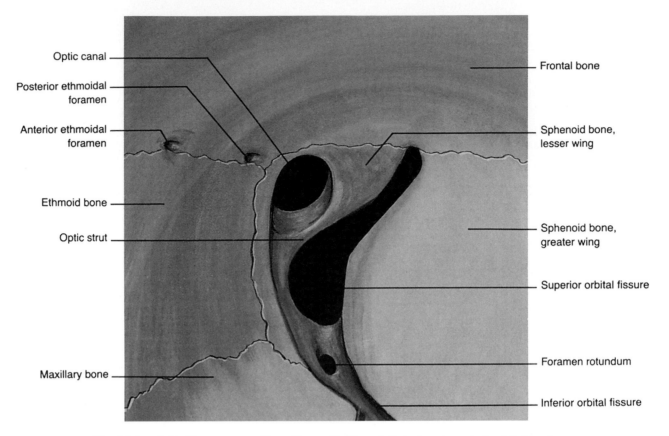

Fig. 10-2   Orbital bones, apex. (From Dutton JJ: *Atlas of clinical and surgical orbital anatomy,* Philadelphia, 1994, WB Saunders.) (See color plate.)

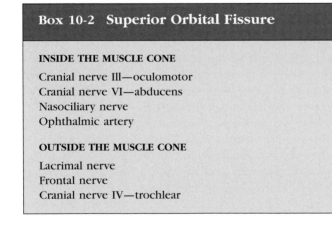

Box 10-2   Superior Orbital Fissure

INSIDE THE MUSCLE CONE

Cranial nerve III—oculomotor
Cranial nerve VI—abducens
Nasociliary nerve
Ophthalmic artery

OUTSIDE THE MUSCLE CONE

Lacrimal nerve
Frontal nerve
Cranial nerve IV—trochlear

Box 10-3   Innervation of the Extraocular Muscles

CRANIAL NERVE III (OCULOMOTOR)
Superior Division

Superior rectus
Levator palpebrae superioris

Inferior Division

Medial rectus
Inferior rectus
Inferior oblique

CRANIAL NERVE IV (TROCHLEAR)

Superior oblique

CRANIAL NERVE VI (ABDUCENS)

Lateral rectus

rolaterally, under the superior rectus, to insert on the globe superiorly.

The oblique muscles attach posterior to the equator of the eye. Their primary action is torsional, although both have a vertical action also. The superior oblique muscle lowers the eye and the inferior oblique raises it; these effects are most pronounced with the eye directed medially.

The extraocular muscles have an unusual microscopic structure. They are a mixture of two distinctly different types of striated muscle fiber, the fibrillenstruktur, or fast twitch, and the felderstruktur fiber, which contracts more slowly and smoothly. The fibrillenstruktur fibers are similar to those of other striated muscle, but the feldenstruktur fibers in mammals are found only in ex-

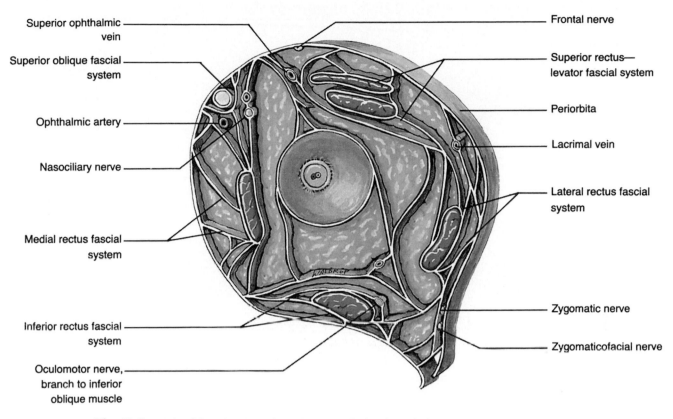

Superior ophthalmic vein
Superior oblique fascial system
Ophthalmic artery
Nasociliary nerve
Medial rectus fascial system
Inferior rectus fascial system
Oculomotor nerve, branch to inferior oblique muscle

Frontal nerve
Superior rectus—levator fascial system
Periorbita
Lacrimal vein
Lateral rectus fascial system
Zygomatic nerve
Zygomaticofacial nerve

Fig. 10-3   Orbital fascial system, frontal view, midorbit through the posterior pole of the globe. (From Dutton JJ: *Atlas of clinical and surgical orbital anatomy*, Philadelphia, 1994, WB Saunders.) (See color plate.)

traocular muscle. These two different muscle fiber types probably explain saccadic movement and slow pursuit, respectively.

The extraocular muscles also have the highest ratio of nerve endings to muscle fibers, about one nerve fiber per three or fewer muscle fibers. This ratio contrasts markedly with that of skeletal muscle elsewhere in the body, with more than 100 muscle fibers per nerve ending. Such an abundance of neural connections allows for fine control and coordination.

FASCIA

We tend to think of the eye as being cushioned in the orbit by adipose tissue. This is true, but the adipose tissue is not simply disorganized "filler." Many connective tissue fascia act as a suspensory system, not only for the globe, but also for the muscles and vessels of the eye (Fig. 10-3), both supporting these structures and limiting their movement. Adipose tissue fills the spaces in between the fascial planes. The muscles are joined by the intermuscular septum, which divides the extraconal from the intraconal space.

The fascia closest to the globe is Tenon's capsule, which surrounds the eye from limbus to optic nerve. It fuses to the limbus just beneath the conjunctiva and also at the optic nerve and is pierced by the muscles posterior to the equator to attach to the globe. Tenon's capsule acts as a space between the globe and the orbital fat, suspending the eye. The muscles are joined by the intermuscular septum, which divides the extraconal from the intraconal space.

NERVES AND CILIARY GANGLION

Most of the sensory and motor nerves enter the orbit through the superior orbital fissure (see Box 10-2). Some, such as cranial nerves III and VI and also the nasociliary branch of cranial nerve V, enter within the annulus of Zinn. Others enter superior to the extraocular muscles, including the lacrimal and frontal nerves, which also originate from the ophthalmic branch of cranial nerve V; and cranial nerve IV (Fig. 10-4).

The ciliary ganglion is located temporal to the optic nerve, close to the orbital apex. Parasympathetic fibers en route to the iris and ciliary body synapse here, whereas sympathetic fibers and fibers from the ophthalmic division of cranial nerve V pass through without synapsing.

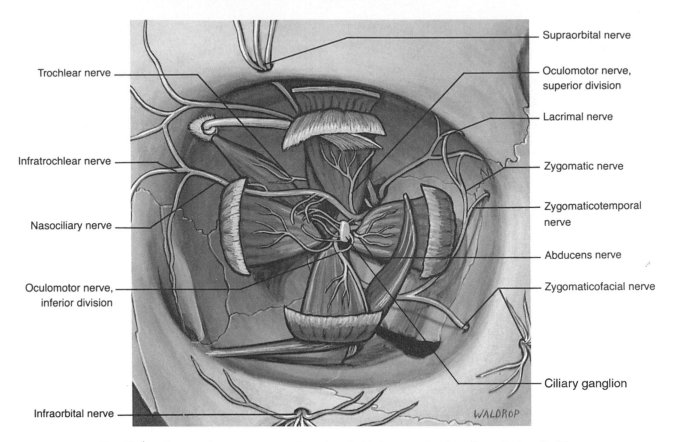

Fig. 10-4   Motor and sensory nerves, frontal periorbital composite view. (From Dutton JJ: *Atlas of clinical and surgical orbital anatomy,* Philadelphia, 1994, WB Saunders.) (See color plate.)

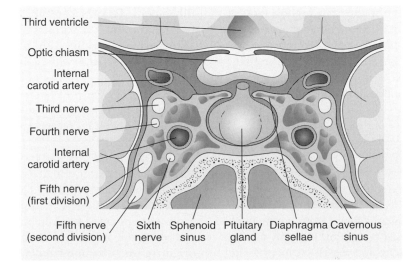

Fig. 10-5   Coronal section through the optic chiasm and cavernous sinuses. The chiasm is flanked laterally by the supraclinoid segments of the carotid arteries and inferolaterally by the cavernous sinuses through which pass the oculomotor nerves and first two division of the trigeminal nerve. (Adapted from Warwick R, editor: Eugene Wolff's anatomy of the eye and orbit, ed 7, Philadelphia, 1976, WB Saunders. In Yanoff M, Duker JS: *Ophthalmology,* St Louis, 1999, Mosby.) (See color plate.)

MAJOR POINTS

The bony orbit borders the frontal lobe of the brain, and the ethmoid, sphenoid, frontal, and maxillary sinuses.

The optic nerve exits the orbit through the optic canal.

The superior orbital fissure is a conduit for several structures, including nerves to the extraocular muscles and the ophthalmic artery.

The extraocular muscles and levator muscle originate at the orbital apex, forming a fascial ring surrounding the optic nerve. The inferior oblique does not participate in this ring, instead originating medially in the orbit.

The horizontal rectus muscles move the eye horizontally. The vertical rectus and the oblique muscles have both vertical and rotational components to their actions.

All four rectus muscles insert anterior to the equator. The two oblique muscles insert posteriorly.

The macula underlies the attachment of the inferior oblique muscle.

The orbital fascia acts to connect the muscles together and to form a suspension system for the globe in the orbit.

Parasympathetic fibers synapse in the ciliary ganglion. The ganglion is also a conduit for sympathetic fibers and fibers from the first division of the trigeminal nerve (cranial nerve V), which pass through without synapsing.

The ophthalmic artery supplies the globe and orbit via its branches. The eye and orbit drain by means of the superior and inferior ophthalmic veins.

The cavernous sinus acts as a conduit for the internal carotid artery and cranial nerves III, IV, VI, and the first two divisions of V.

BLOOD SUPPLY

The major artery of the orbit and indeed of the eye itself is the ophthalmic artery. The internal carotid artery enters the cranial cavity through the foramen lacerum and then enters the cavernous sinus, along with cranial nerve VI. There it gives off its first branch, the ophthalmic artery, which enters the orbit through the superior orbital fissure.

The orbital veins do not parallel the arteries. Veins from the orbit, globe, and face exit via the superior and inferior ophthalmic veins to drain into the cavernous sinus.

The cavernous sinus is a venous sinus that lies immediately behind the superior orbital fissure and beneath the chiasm (Fig. 10-5). Not only is it the major venous drain for the orbital and facial vessels, but it also acts as a conduit for the internal carotid artery and for cranial nerves III, IV, VI, and the first two divisions of cranial nerve V. All of these are attached to the lateral wall of the sinus except for cranial nerve VI.

SUGGESTED READINGS

Clark RA, Miller JM, Demer JL: Location and stability of rectus muscle pulleys: muscle paths as a function of gaze, *Invest Ophthalmol Vis Sci* 38:227-240, 1997.

Demer JL, Miller JM: Magnetic resonance imaging of the functional anatomy of the superior oblique muscle, *Invest Ophthalmol Vis Sci* 36:906-913, 1995.

Ettl A, Kramer J, Daxer A, Koornneef L: High resolution magnetic resonance imaging of neurovascular orbital anatomy, *Ophthalmology* 104:869-877, 1997.

Goldberg RA, Hannani K, Toga AW: Microanatomy of the orbital apex: computer tomography and microcryoplaning of soft and hard tissue, *Ophthalmology* 99:1447-1452, 1992.

Goldberg RA, Kim AJ, Kerivan KM: The lacrimal keyhole, orbital door jamb, and basin of the inferior orbital fissure: three areas of deep bone in the lateral orbit, *Arch Ophthalmol* 116:1618-1624, 1998.

Williamson TH, Harris A: Color Doppler ultrasound imaging of the eye and orbit, *Surv Ophthalmol* 40:255-267, 1996.

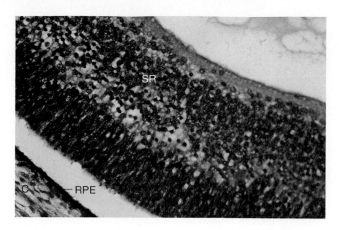

Plate 2-10

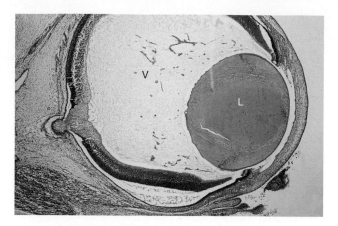

Plate 2-11

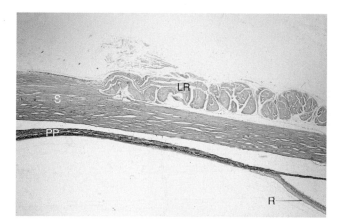

Plate 3-4

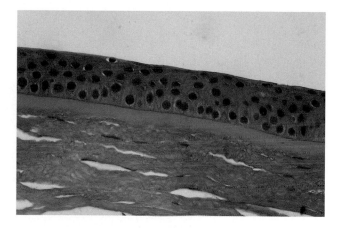

Plate 4-1

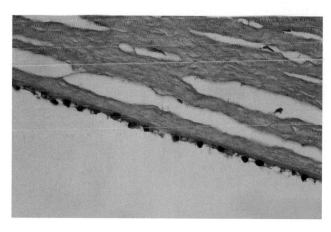

Plate 4-5

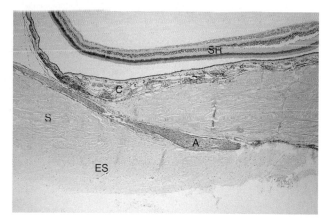

Plate 4-8

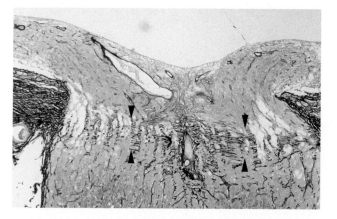

Plate 4-9

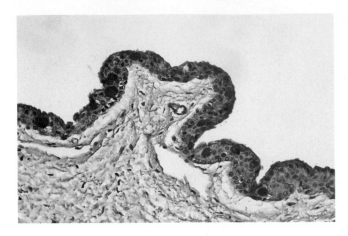

Plate 5-2

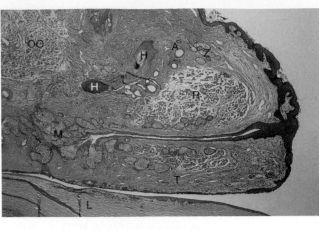

Plate 5-5

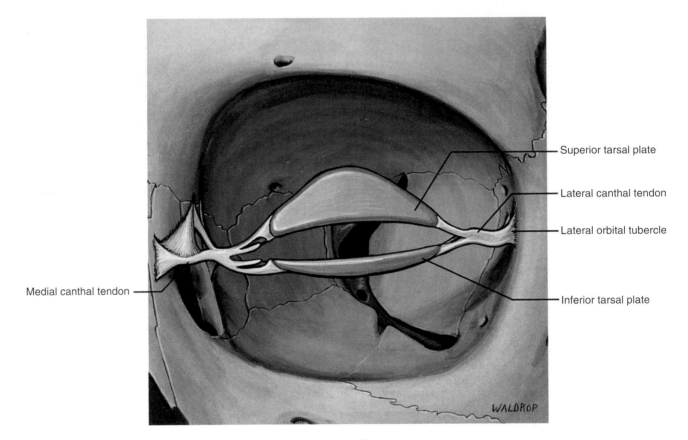

Superior tarsal plate

Lateral canthal tendon

Lateral orbital tubercle

Medial canthal tendon

Inferior tarsal plate

WALDROP

Plate 5-6

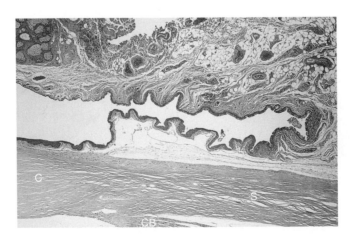

Plate 5-7

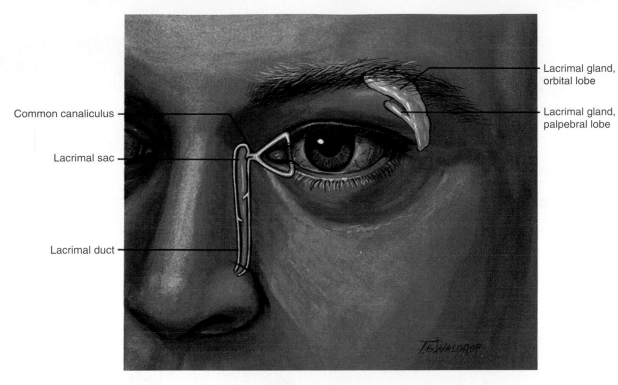

Common canaliculus

Lacrimal sac

Lacrimal duct

Lacrimal gland, orbital lobe

Lacrimal gland, palpebral lobe

Platc 5-8

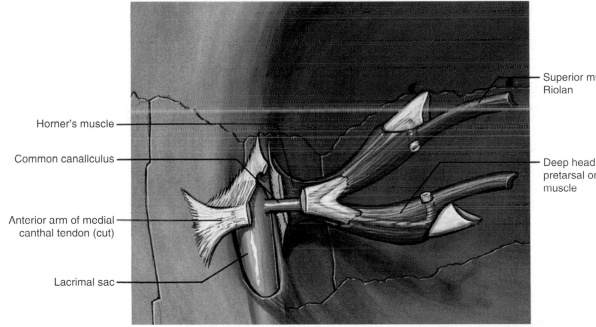

Horner's muscle

Common canallculus

Anterior arm of medial canthal tendon (cut)

Lacrimal sac

Superior muscle of Riolan

Deep head of inferior pretarsal orbicularis muscle

Plate 5-9

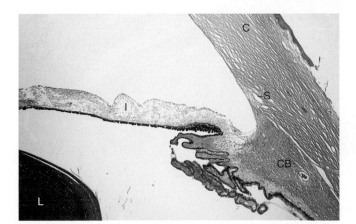

Plate 6-1

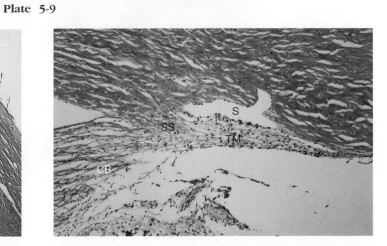

Plate 6-4

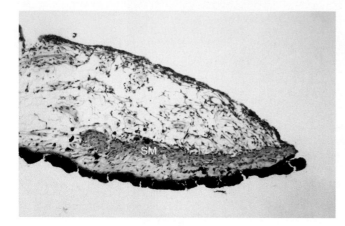

Plate 7-3

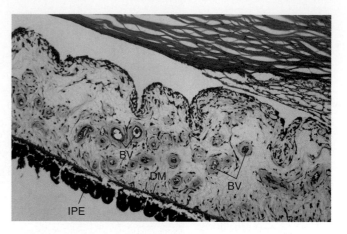

Plate 7-5

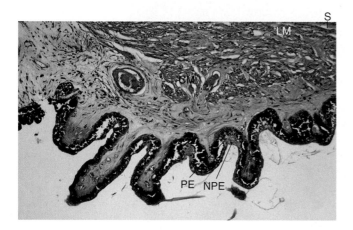

Plate 7-6

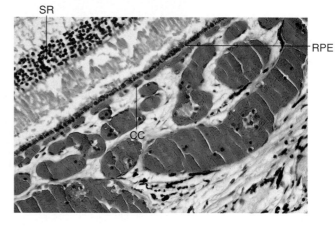

Plate 7-8

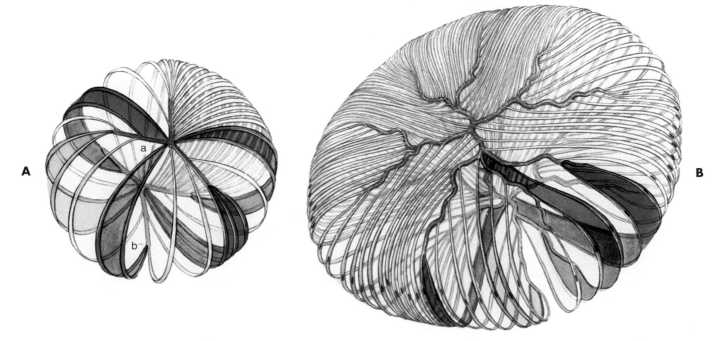

Plate 8-4 A and B

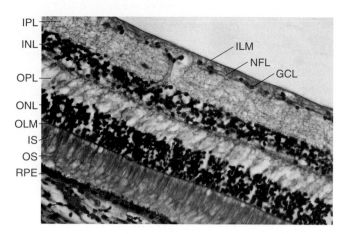

IPL
INL
OPL
ONL
OLM
IS
OS
RPE

ILM
NFL
GCL

Plate 9-2

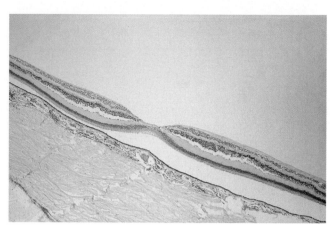

Plate 9-10

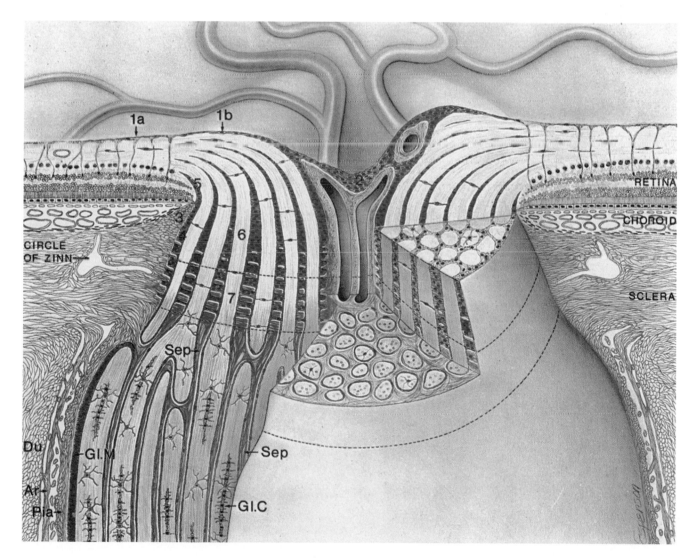

1a
1b

5
3
4
6
7

RETINA
CHOROID

CIRCLE OF ZINN

SCLERA

Sep

Du
Ar
Pia

Gl.M
Sep
Gl.C

Plate 9-13

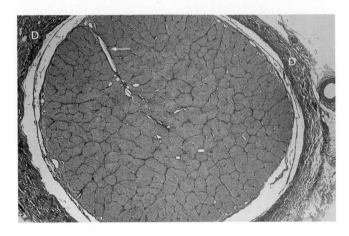

Plate 9-14

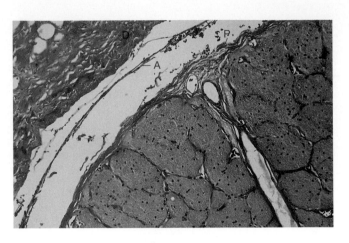

Plate 9-15

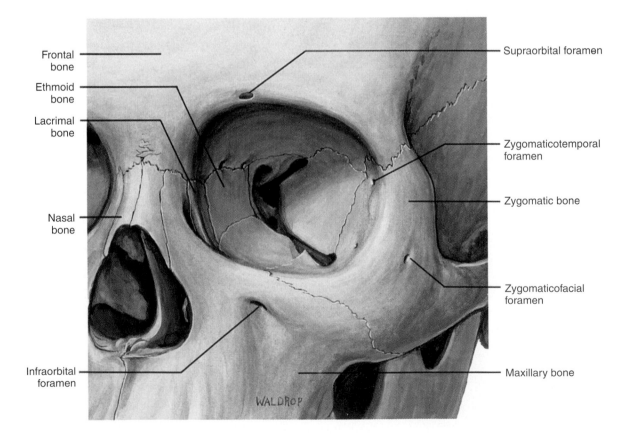

Frontal bone

Ethmoid bone

Lacrimal bone

Nasal bone

Infraorbital foramen

Supraorbital foramen

Zygomaticotemporal foramen

Zygomatic bone

Zygomaticofacial foramen

Maxillary bone

WALDROP

Plate 10-01

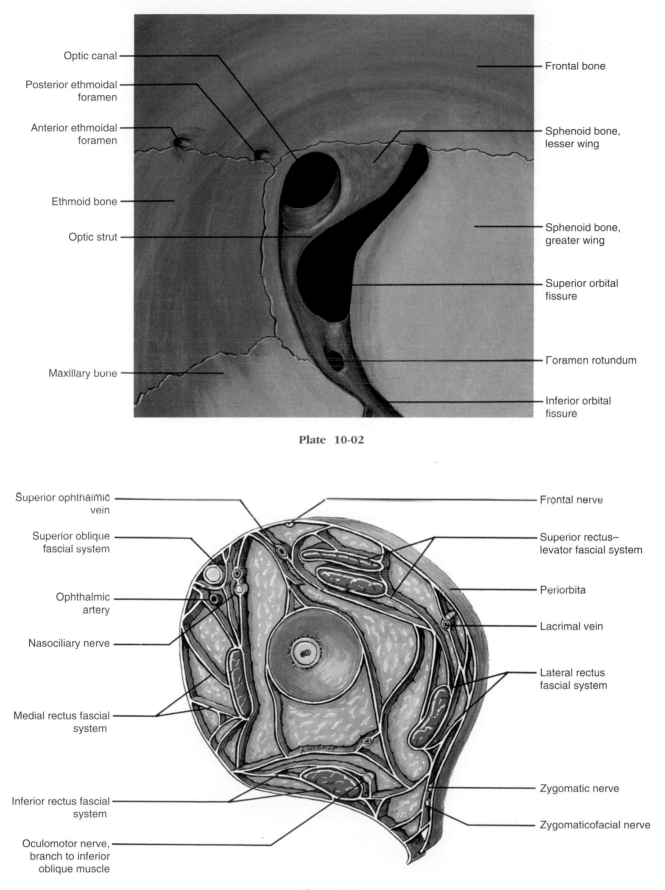

Optic canal

Posterior ethmoidal
foramen

Anterior ethmoidal
foramen

Ethmoid bone

Optic strut

Maxillary bone

Frontal bone

Sphenoid bone,
lesser wing

Sphenoid bone,
greater wing

Superior orbital
fissure

Foramen rotundum

Inferior orbital
fissure

Plate 10-02

Superior ophthalmic
vein

Superior oblique
fascial system

Ophthalmic
artery

Nasociliary nerve

Medial rectus fascial
system

Inferior rectus fascial
system

Oculomotor nerve,
branch to inferior
oblique muscle

Frontal nerve

Superior rectus–
levator fascial system

Periorbita

Lacrimal vein

Lateral rectus
fascial system

Zygomatic nerve

Zygomaticofacial nerve

Plate 10-03

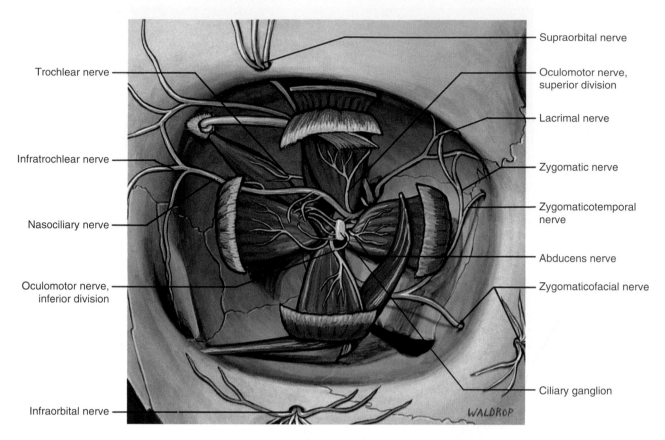

Supraorbital nerve

Trochlear nerve

Oculomotor nerve, superior division

Lacrimal nerve

Infratrochlear nerve

Zygomatic nerve

Zygomaticotemporal nerve

Nasociliary nerve

Abducens nerve

Zygomaticofacial nerve

Oculomotor nerve, inferior division

Ciliary ganglion

Infraorbital nerve

Plate 10-04

OPTIC CHIASM AND CAVERNOUS SINUSES (CORONAL SECTION)

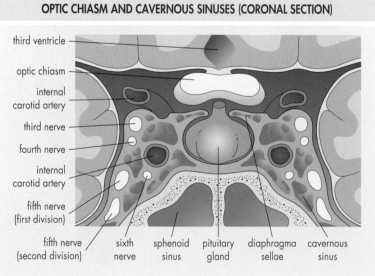

third ventricle

optic chiasm

internal carotid artery

third nerve

fourth nerve

internal carotid artery

fifth nerve (first division)

fifth nerve (second division)

sixth nerve

sphenoid sinus

pituitary gland

diaphragma sellae

cavernous sinus

Plate 10-05

REFRACTION

CONSTANCE E. WEST

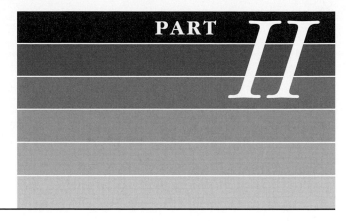

PART *II*

CHAPTER 11

Ophthalmic Optics

This chapter introduces ophthalmic optics, a framework for describing and quantifying the behavior of light in an optical system.

REFRACTIVE INDEX

Light slows down when it encounters a refractive medium (Fig. 11-1). The refractive index of a transparent material is the ratio of the speed of light in a vacuum to the speed of light in that material:

$$\text{Refractive index} = n_{\text{material}} = \text{speed of light in a vacuum/speed of light in material.}$$

Because light always travels faster in a vacuum, *no* material has an index of refraction less than 1.000. The indices of refraction for commonly encountered ophthalmic materials are listed in Table 11-1.

SNELL'S LAW

Snell's law governs the refraction, or bending, of light rays as they travel from one medium to another. The interface between the media is called the refracting surface. Snell's law quantifies how strongly light rays are bent when they pass from one medium to another. The amount of bending is compared to an imaginary line drawn perpendicular to the refracting surface called the *normal.* When light travels from a material with a lower index of refraction to one with a higher index, the light is bent toward the normal (Fig. 11-2). Conversely, when light travels from a material with a higher index of refraction to one with a lower index, the light is bent away from the normal (Fig. 11-3). When a ray of light strikes the refracting surface perpendicularly, it does not change direction, but it does speed up (the new material has a lower index of refraction) or slow down (the new material has a higher index of refraction). The exact amount of refraction, or bending, is determined by Snell's law:

$$n \sin i = n' \sin r',$$

where n and n' are the indices of refraction, i is the angle of the light relative to the normal, and r is the angle of the refracted ray relative to the normal (Fig. 11-4). One can think of this qualitatively as a material with a higher index of refraction being harder for the light to get through, so the light has to take a shorter path through the material. The sine values for selected angles, in degrees, are listed in Table 11-2.

The speed of light in a material depends not only upon the index of refraction of the material, but also upon the wavelength of the light; technically, each wavelength has a unique index of refraction for a given medium. The index of refraction listed in ophthalmic textbooks is for sodium (yellow) light with a wavelength of 589 nm.

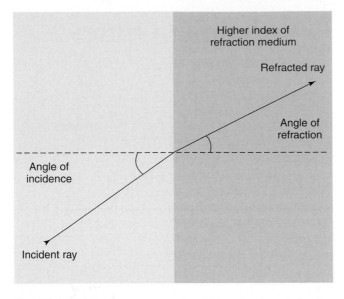

Fig. 11-1 Light slows down when it encounters a refractive medium. When it travels from a medium with a lower index of refraction to one with a higher index of refraction, rays are bent toward the normal.

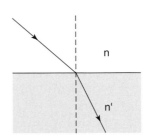

Fig. 11-2 When light travels from a media with a lower index of refraction to one with a higher index of refraction, the light is bent toward the normal.

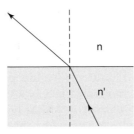

Fig. 11-3 When light travels from a material with a higher index of refraction to one with a lower index, the light is bent away from the normal.

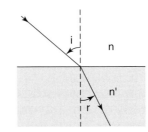

Fig. 11-4 The incident ray, the normal, and the refracted ray all lie in the same plane. The angle of the incident ray relative to the normal is *i*, and the angle of the refracted ray relative to the normal is *r*.

Table 11-1	Refractive indices of common ophthalmic materials
Material	**Refractive index**
Air	1.00
Aqueous, vitreous	1.34
Keratometric	1.3375
Cornea	1.37
Crystalline lens	1.42
Crown glass	1.52
Polycarbonate	1.59
Plastic (PMMA, CR-39)	Up to 1.66
High-index glass	Up to 1.81

Table 11-2	Sine table
Angle (degrees)	**Sine**
0	0.000
10	0.174
20	0.342
30	0.500
40	0.643
50	0.766
60	0.866
70	0.940
80	0.985
90	1.000

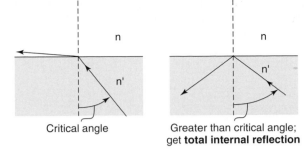

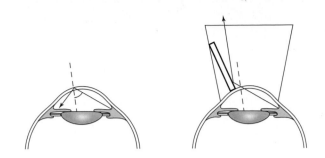

Fig. 11-5 Critical angle. Total internal reflection can happen only when light passes from a medium with a higher index of refraction to a media with a lower one. The critical angle is the angle at which light ceases to be refracted and is internally reflected.

Fig. 11-6 Gonioprisms replace the tear/air interface with glass or plastic, and use a mirror to reflect the rays in order to view angle structures.

CRITICAL ANGLE AND TOTAL INTERNAL REFLECTION

Definition

When a light ray travels from a medium with a higher index of refraction to one with a lower index, total internal reflection is possible. Total internal reflection can *only* happen when light passes from a material with a *higher* index of refraction to a material with a *lower* one. The critical angle is the angle at which light ceases to be refracted and is internally reflected (Fig. 11-5). The critical angle can be calculated by determining the incident angle that causes the refracted angle (relative to the normal) to be 90°:

$$n \sin i = n' \sin 90°.$$

Because the sine of 90° is 1.00, the equation can be rearranged to

$$\sin i = n'/n$$
$$i = \text{arc sin } (n'/n).$$

The critical angle for crown glass is 41°, and for tear film it is 49°. Total internal reflection is important in many areas of ophthalmology and surgical instrumentation, as discussed next under "Clinical Applications."

Clinical Applications

Because of total internal reflection, light emerging from the angle of the anterior segment is reflected back into the eye; the angle structures are not directly visible to the clinician. Total internal reflection is obviated by goniolenses to view the angle structures (Fig. 11-6). The mirrored types of goniolenses replace air with plastic or glass and use a mirror to reflect the rays to form an *indirect* view of the angle. A Koeppe goniolens also replaces the air with plastic, but has a highly curved anterior sur-

Box 11-1 Total Internal Reflection in Ophthalmology

Fiberoptic light sources
Goniolenses
Eye pieces of indirect ophthalmoscope
Outer segments of photoreceptors

face that allows the light rays from the angle to strike the Koeppe lens/air surface at less than the critical angle and allows the observer to have a *direct* view of the angle.

If the cornea is very steep (as in some patients with keratoconus) or its diameter is very large (e.g., occasional patients with congenital glaucoma who have a clear cornea or housecats), the light leaving the eye may strike the tear/air interface at less than the critical angle. In this case the angle structures may be visible on direct inspection without the aid of a goniolens.

Total internal reflection can be used to our advantage in ophthalmic instruments. Surgical headlights and endoscopic light sources use fiberoptic cables that transmit light through a bundle of glass fibers. The light ricochets off the sides of each fiber as it is totally internally reflected down the length of the cable; this results in very efficient light propagation with very little light loss. When the glass fibers in the cable become broken, the amount of light produced is reduced. Some indirect ophthalmoscopes use prisms in the eyepieces to optically collapse the interpupillary diameter. There is total internal reflection of the light in the prism so that there is very little light loss.

Total internal reflection may also play a part in the retina, where the outer segments of the rods and cones are thought to "trap" the incident light via total internal reflection. The applications of total internal reflection in ophthalmology are summarized in Box 11-1.

VERGENCE

Definition

Vergence is an important concept and is used primarily in ophthalmic optics. It is a measure of the coming together or spreading apart of a bundle of light rays as it comes from (or toward) a single point, as shown in Fig. 11-7. By definition, a bundle of light rays coming together has positive (plus) vergence, and bundle spreading apart has negative (minus) vergence. Bundles of light rays that are parallel have zero vergence. If light rays from an extended object (one that has many, many points) have zero vergence, the light is said to be collimated (Table 11-3). Rays from real points diverge and therefore have minus vergence. Rays that are converging (positive vergence) have generally been created by an optical system.

Vergence is an extremely useful concept, because it allows calculation of the location of an image formed by an optical system. Some teachers of ophthalmic optics stress the use of sign conventions to locate and orient an image relative to its object. The author prefers that the reader not get confused by sign conventions, but rather tries to understand the overall contribution of a lens to a system by whether it adds to or subtracts from the vergence of the optical system, and therefore whether it pulls the image toward the lens or pushes it away from the lens.

Diopter

A diopter is the unit that quantifies vergence. It is the reciprocal of the distance (in meters) from the point where the light rays would intersect if extended in either direction (Fig. 11-8). As the distance from the point becomes smaller, the negative or positive vergence becomes greater.

Lenses alter the vergence of light by causing the entering light rays to come together (adding plus vergence) or to spread apart (adding minus vergence). The amount of vergence contributed by a lens is measured in diopters. A given lens contributes a specified amount of vergence to the system, regardless of whether the light entering the lens has positive (light rays coming together), negative (light rays spreading apart), or zero (light rays parallel) vergence.

The Basic Lens Formula

The basic lens formula, or vergence formula, is one of the few formulas the clinician must know. It is

$$U + D = V$$

where U is the vergence of light entering the system, D is the amount of vergence contributed by the lens, and V is the vergence of light exiting the lens. U, D, and V are measured in diopters. The basic lens (vergence) formula is used to determine the location of objects and images as discussed later in this chapter.

Table 11-3	Vergence definitions
Positive	Light rays coming together
Negative	Light rays spreading apart
Zero	Light rays parallel
Collimated	Light rays from an extended object that have zero vergence

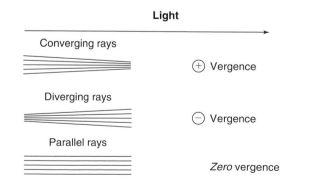

Fig. 11-7 Vergence is a measure of the coming together or spreading apart of a bundle of light rays.

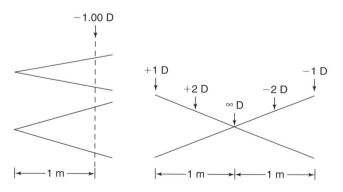

Fig. 11-8 Diopters are the unit of measurement of vergence. It is the reciprocal of the distance (in meters) from the point where the light rays would intersect if extended in either direction. The smaller the distance from the point, the greater the vergence. The vergence is infinite where the light rays intersect.

FOCAL POINTS AND LENGTHS

An ideal, thin lens can be described by the location of its focal point. In ophthalmic optics, each lens has a primary and a secondary focal point.

The primary focal point of a lens is the point along the optical axis at which an object must be placed for parallel rays to emerge from the lens and form an image at infinity (Fig. 11-9). The secondary focal point of a lens is that point along the optical axis where parallel incident rays are brought to a focus.

An easy way to remember the location of the primary and secondary focal points of a plus and minus lens follows. Consider light rays from the sun with (almost) zero vergence that are incident on a common household magnifying lens (a plus lens). An ant (or a piece of paper) that is placed at the lens' secondary focal point will be warmed (or burned!). Burning ants in this manner is "second nature" to some school children—and it happens because they are placing the ant at the secondary focal point of the lens.

The focal length of a lens is the distance from the ideal thin lens to its focal point and is measured in meters. The focal length (in meters) is equal to the reciprocal of the dioptric power of the lens:

$$D_{lens} = 1/\text{focal length}$$

or

$$\text{Focal length (meters)} = 1/D_{lens}$$

Thus a 4 D lens has a focal length of 0.25 m (25 cm), and a lens with a focal length of 10 cm had a power of 10 D.

When one works optics problems, it is very useful to be able to readily convert diopters to focal length and focal length to diopters without manual calculation. Table 11-4 provides these values, and the author strongly suggests that the reader become familiar with them to more easily work on optics problems.

USING THE BASIC LENS (VERGENCE) FORMULA TO LOCATE AN IMAGE

Using the vergence formula, one can locate the position of an image. Consider an object located 2 m to the left of a +2 D lens (Fig.11-10). The vergence entering the lens is −1/2 = −0.5 D (negative vergence because the light rays are diverging from the object). The lens adds 2 D of positive vergence. Thus the vergence exiting the lens is −0.5 + 2 = +1.5 D. Light leaving the lens with a convergence of +1.5 D will come to a point 1/1.5 = 0.67 m from the lens.

Objects and images can be located on opposite sides of the lens, as seen in Fig. 11-10, or on the same side of the lens, as seen in Fig. 11-11.

Table 11-4 Dioptric power and focal length

Power (D)	Focal length (cm)
0.5	200
1.0	100
1.5	67
2.0	50
2.5	40
3	33
4	25
5	20
6	16.7
7	14
8	12.5
9	11
10	10
11	9
12	8.3
15	6.7
20	5

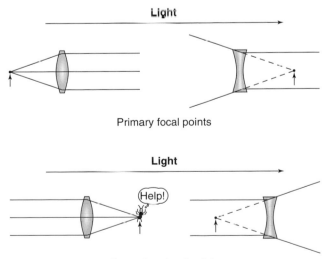

Fig. 11-9   The primary and secondary focal points of plus and minus lenses.

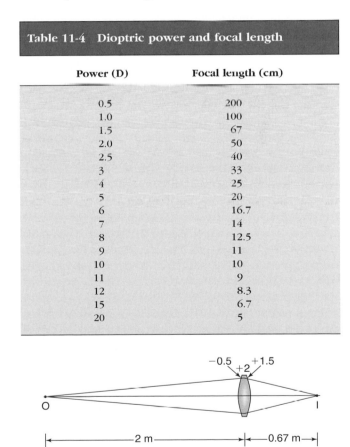

Fig. 11-10   An object is located 2 m to the left of a +2.00 D lens. The vergence of the light leaving the lens is +1.5 D.

OBJECTS AND IMAGES: REAL OR VIRTUAL?

The object *rays* in an optical system are on the incoming side of the lens, and the image *rays* are located on the outgoing side of the lens (Fig. 11-12). Consider a lens system in which the object is located on the same side of the lens as the object rays; this object is real. An object located on the side of the lens opposite to its object rays is virtual. Virtual objects (or images) are lo-

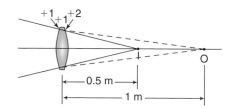

Fig. 11-11   A virtual object forms a real image in this illustration, and both are located to the right of the lens.

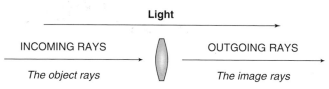

Fig. 11-12   The object rays are located on the incoming side of the lens, and the image rays are located on the outgoing side of the lens.

cated through imaginary extensions of the object (or image) rays through the lens (Fig. 11-13).

An alternative way to conceptualize the issue of real/virtual objects/images is to asses whether the object (or image) rays are converging or diverging as they enter (or exit) the lens. Consider the object and its rays first. When rays entering the lens are divergent, the object is real; when the rays entering are convergent, the object must be virtual. Now consider the image and its rays. When the rays exiting the lens are convergent, the image is real; when the light exiting the lens is divergent, the image must be virtual (Fig. 11-13).

THE CENTRAL RAY: IMAGE SIZE AND ORIENTATION

In ophthalmic optics problems it is often necessary to determine not only the location, but also the size and orientation of the image relative to the object. Whereas the images formed by mirrors and lenses are *located* along the optical axis using the vergence formula ($U + D = V$) introduced previously in this chapter, simple ray tracing can be used to help define the size and orientation of the image. Many students of ophthalmic optics find ray-tracing exercises tedious, but the "central ray" is a simple and valuable tool to assist in determining the size and orientation of the image. The central ray passes from the tip of the object through the center of the lens and extends infinitely far in both directions, as shown in Fig. 11-14.

The intersection of the central ray with the image plane (located using the vergence formula) locates the

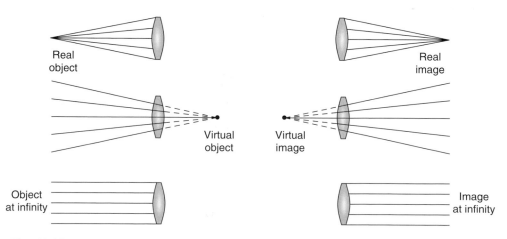

Fig. 11-13   A virtual object (or image) is located through an imaginary extension of the object (or image) rays through the lens.

tip of the image. The corresponding points of the object and its image must always fall on the central ray. This allows the student to visually determine whether the image is upright or inverted. Consider the examples shown in Fig. 11-15. In the *top portion* of the figure, an inverted image is formed by a plus lens; the location of the object is determined using the vergence formula. Using the central ray concept, one can see that images on the same side of the lens as the object have the same orientation as the object. Those formed on the opposite side of the lens are inverted relative to the object.

Remember that objects are not always real, as discussed earlier in this chapter. Consider the possible images that can be formed with a virtual object, as shown in Fig. 11-15, *bottom*. A virtual object can form erect, real images or inverted, virtual images, depending on the vergence of the light entering the lens and of the lens power itself.

Using similar triangles formed by the central ray and the object and image, one can graphically show how large or small the image is with respect to the object and what its orientation is. The sizes of the object and its image depend upon the distances of each of them from the lens. The farther away from the lens an object or image is, the larger it is. The key steps in determining the properties of an object and image are summarized in Box 11-2.

MULTIPLE LENS SYSTEMS

When a multiple lens system is analyzed, the central rays are drawn in succession for each object/lens/image combination as shown in Fig. 11-16. The image formed by the first lens becomes the object for the second lens, and the image formed by the second lens becomes the object for the third lens, and so on. One should always determine the vergence entering the lens using the distance from where the rays *would have* intersected.

Box 11-2 Key Steps in Determining the Properties of an Object and Image

Images and objects are *located* along the optical axis using the vergence formula ($U + D = V$).

The relative *size* is determined by the ratio of the distances of the image and the object from the lens (image size/object size).

The *orientation* (upright/inverted) is determined using the central ray concept.

An object/image is *real* if it is located on the same side of the lens as its respective rays, and *virtual* if it is on the opposite side.

For multiple lens systems, each lens and its object-image pair are considered separately. The image of the preceding lens serves as the object for the next lens (see text).

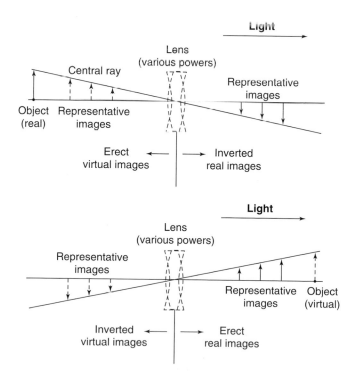

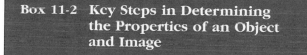

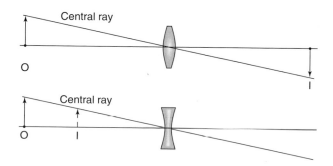

Fig. 11-14   The central ray passes from the tip of the object through the center of the lens and extends infinitely far in both directions.

Fig. 11-15   Using the central ray to determine image and object size and orientation. A real object is shown in the top figure with representative images, depending on the location of the image. A virtual object is shown in the bottom of the figure with the central ray helping to determine the size and orientation of the possible images.

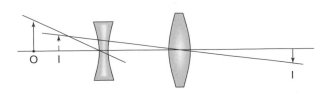

Fig. 11-16 Using the central ray in optical systems with multiple lenses, the central ray is drawn for each object/lens/image combination in succession. The image formed by the preceding lens becomes the object for the next lens.

Light →

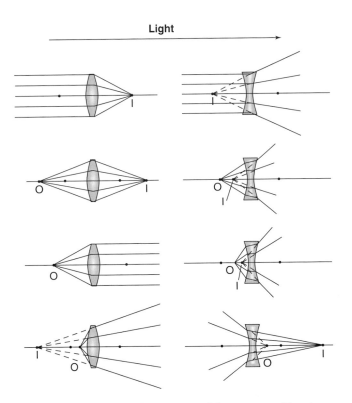

Fig. 11-17 When an object is moved from one position to another in an optical system, the image moves in the same direction.

OBJECT AND IMAGE MOVEMENT

When an object is moved from one position to another in an optical system, the image will also move. How far does the image move and which way?

The image always moves in the same direction as the object moves relative to the light, as shown in Fig. 11-17. The image usually does not move the same distance as the object does, but it *always* moves in the same direction. If the object moves to the right, the image moves to the right.

This principle of object and image movement has practical implications in ophthalmic practice. If an ob-

ject is in focus on the retina and it is pushed closer to the eye, the image is pushed in the same direction (behind the retina!) unless the eye can accommodate to focus the image again. If an object is moved beyond the far point of a myopic eye, the image is pulled in the same direction—off the retina and into the vitreous. In the operating room, moving the microscope up "pulls" its focal point with it and relaxes the accommodation of the surgeon.

Image movement can also be accomplished by the addition of lenses into the optical system.

REFRACTION BY CURVED SURFACE

Snell's law can be used to calculate the amount of refraction of light that occurs at a surface. Snell's law deals with the refraction of light relative to a line drawn perpendicular (normal) to the surface. However, most optical elements (like a lens or the cornea) have a curved surface. By using small angle approximations and considering paraxial rays (those close to the optical axis of the system) only, the power of a spherical refracting surface can be mathematically derived. The derivation of this equation is beyond the scope of this introductory text, but it states that the power of the surface, $D_{surface}$, is

$$D_{surface} = |n - n'|/r$$

where $|n - n'|$ is the difference in the refractive indices of the two materials and r is the radius of curvature of the surface in meters. Thus the power of a spherical refracting surface is *directly* proportional to the difference in refractive index and *inversely* proportional to the curvature of the surface. The dioptric power of a surface becomes greater if there is a greater difference in refractive index between the two materials or if the surface has a smaller radius of curvature.

The sign of the power can be easily determined by considering the shape of a lens formed by the material with the *higher* refractive index (Fig. 11-18). Start by drawing a rectangle around the curved surface. If the shape of the "lens" formed by the material with the higher refractive index is planoconcave, the surface has minus power. If it has a convex shape, it has plus power.

Clinical Application

The front surface of the cornea has plus power and adds convergence to incoming light rays. The back surface of the cornea, however, has minus power because the material with the higher refractive index (the cornea)

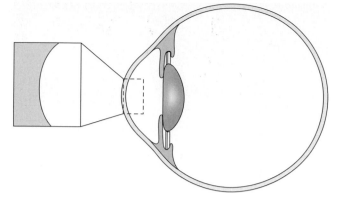

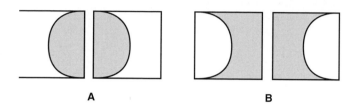

Fig. 11-18 Refraction by a curved surface. Draw a rectangle around the curved surface, and determine the "shape" of the material with the higher index of refraction. If the "shape" of the lens formed by the media with the higher index of refraction is planoconvex **(A)**, the surface has plus power. Conversely, if the "shape" of the lens formed by the media with the higher index of refraction is planoconcave **(B)**, the surface has minus power.

Fig. 11-19 The posterior surface of the cornea has minus power, because it has the higher index of refraction and is concave.

is concave, as shown in Fig. 11-19. The back surface of the cornea, therefore, diverges the light rays. Overall, however, the cornea is considered to have plus power because the difference in refractive index between the cornea and air (1.37 − 1.00, anterior corneal surface) is far greater than the difference between the cornea and aqueous (1.37 − 1.33, posterior surface). Most refractive surgery relies upon altering the curvature of the anterior surface of the cornea to change the dioptric power of the central cornea.

SUGGESTED READING

Guyton DL, West CE, Miller JM, Wisnicki HJ: *Ophthalmic optics,* Baltimore, 1999, Prism Press

Ogle KN: *Optics,* Springfield IL, 1968, Charles C Thomas.

Thick Lenses and Models of the Human Eye

Only an *ideal* lens can be described by just the location of its optical center and two focal points. A *real* lens is described by its cardinal points, to be discussed in this chapter. An optical system that is composed of real lenses (including mirrors) and differing refractive indices can be *reduced,* or simplified mathematically, using Gaussian optics, to a single lens system with two nodal points, two principal planes, and two focal points. Schematic, or model, eyes are useful mathematical constructs of the optical system of the human eye; they are used in optics problems that help one to understand the relative effects of the anatomy of structural lesions of the retina and to design intraocular lenses.

THICK LENSES

An ordinary, real lens is described by the location of its six *cardinal points* as shown in Fig. 12-1: two principal points (H and H'), two nodal points (n and n'), and two focal points (F and F'). The principal points are usually referred to as the principal planes H and H'. The nodal points of a lens coincide with the principal planes unless the refractive index of the media changes from one side of the optical system to the other, as in the eye. Refraction is considered to occur at the principal planes, and the central ray travels toward the first nodal point and emerges from the second nodal point (parallel to its original direction). The true focal lengths of the lens are measured from the principal planes.

Even an optical system composed of multiple elements can be mathematically reduced using these prin-

ciples to two nodal points, two principal planes, and two focal points.

Clinical Application

The concept of back vertex power becomes important when one measures the power of bifocal segments. As will be discussed in Chapter 15, the bifocal segment's power is ground onto the front surface of the spectacle lens. We measure the back vertex power (reciprocal of the back focal length) with a manual lensmeter. Therefore, it is important to reverse the position of the temples on the stage (Fig. 12-2) to properly measure the power of a bifocal. This is even more important for spectacle lenses with higher distance power.

GULLSTRAND MODEL EYE

Allvar Gullstrand (1862-1930) was the Nobel Laureate in Medicine in 1911 for his work on the "dioptics" of the eye and is the only ophthalmologist ever to have won a Nobel Prize. Gullstrand's schematic eye reduced the focusing components of the eye (tear film, cornea, lens, aqueous, and vitreous) to two principal planes and points and two nodal planes and points. In the Gullstrand model eye (Fig. 12-3), the anterior and posterior focal lengths are different because media that surround the cornea and lens—the air and the vitreous—have different refractive indices. This model is too complicated to allow rapid calculations for many clinical problems, however, and its use is not widespread.

REDUCED SCHEMATIC EYE

The reduced schematic eye (Fig. 12-4) is much easier to deal with mathematically than Gullstrand's model eye,

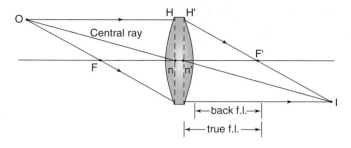

Fig. 12-1   A real lens is described by its six cardinal points: the principal points H and H', the nodal points n and n', and the focal points F and F'. (*f.l.,* focal length.)

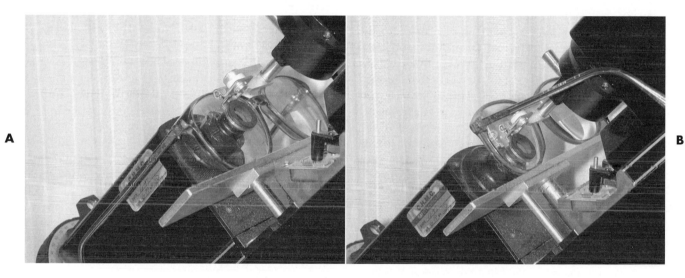

Fig. 12-2   **A,** The distance power of the bifocal glasses is measured with the temples facing away. **B,** Bifocal segments should be measured with the temples oriented toward the clinician.

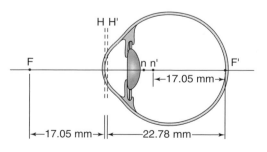

Fig. 12-3   The Gullstrand schematic eye.

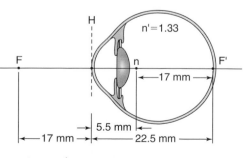

Fig. 12-4   The reduced schematic eye.

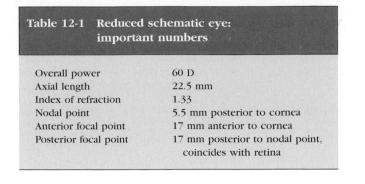

Table 12-1   Reduced schematic eye: important numbers

Overall power	60 D
Axial length	22.5 mm
Index of refraction	1.33
Nodal point	5.5 mm posterior to cornea
Anterior focal point	17 mm anterior to cornea
Posterior focal point	17 mm posterior to nodal point, coincides with retina

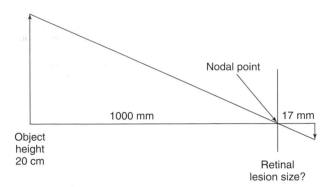

Fig. 12-5   An emmetropic eye has a scotoma 20 cm in diameter on a tangent screen performed one meter from the cornea. The reduced schematic eye and similar triangles can be used to calculate the size of the retinal lesion causing the scotoma (see text; proportions not to scale).

but results are sufficiently accurate for most clinical computations. The reduced schematic eye has only one surface, one nodal point, and one principal plane. The dioptric power of the reduced schematic eye is 60 D and the axial length is 22.5 mm. Refraction is considered to "occur" at the principal plane. The anterior focal point, F, is 17 mm anterior to the principal plane (the cornea). The posterior focal point, which coincides with the retina, is located 17 mm posterior to the nodal point. However, the nodal point does not coincide with the principal plane because the higher refractive index of refraction of the interior of the eye (1.33 in this model) "pushes" the nodal point posteriorly. The nodal point is 5.5 mm posterior to the cornea. This model is quite useful for solving clinical problems involving the eye as an optical system, and the numbers are summarized in Table 12-1. A clinical example follows.

Clinical Application: Calculation of the Size of a Retinal Lesion

The size of a retinal lesion can be calculated from the size of a scotoma on visual field testing, as long as the testing distance is known. Suppose an emmetropic eye has a scotoma 20 cm in diameter on a tangent screen performed 1 m from the cornea (Fig. 12-5). Using the reduced schematic eye and similar triangles, the size of the retinal lesion is 200/1000 = retinal lesion/17. Thus, the diameter of the retinal lesion is 3.4 mm. Although the distance from the cornea to the nodal point can be added into the calculations, the difference is negligible because of the distance of the eye from the tangent screen.

SUGGESTED READING

Rubin ML: *Optics for Clinicians,* ed 3, Gainesville, Fla., 1977, Triad.

CHAPTER 13

The Ametropias

This chapter will address the ametropias, both descriptively and geometrically. Understanding the optical implications of myopia, hyperopia, and emmetropia in terms of geometric optics will help the ophthalmologist to understand common clinical problems including spectacle lenses, contact lenses, intraocular lens implantation, and refractive surgery.

EMMETROPIA

Emmetropia is the lack of a need for refractive correction, such that the power of the optics of the front of the eye (cornea and crystalline lens) is exactly suited for the axial length of the eye. An eye is ametropic when there is a mismatch of the refractive power of the eye and its axial length.

AMETROPIA

Refractive errors, or the ametropias (myopia, hyperopia, and astigmatism), are defined by the location of the secondary focal point/lines of the eye with respect to the retina with accommodation fully relaxed. This is illustrated graphically in Fig. 13-1. Focal points or lines are

never more than a few millimeters from the retina. A general rule of thumb is that each diopter of ametropia pulls the focal point off the retina about ⅓ mm. Thus the secondary focal point of an eye with 3 D myopia is 1 mm in front of the retina, and that for an eye with 3 D hyperopia is 1 mm behind the retina.

Ametropia is due to a "mismatch" of the refractive power of the cornea and lens with the length of the eye. An eye with refractive myopia can be thought of as having an optical system that is too powerful, bringing light rays to a focus in front of the retina. In contrast, an eye with axial myopia has a normal amount of optical power (60 D), but the axial length is too long. In refractive hyperopia, the axial length is normal, but the refractive power of the eye is insufficient to focus the light on the retina. Aphakia is the extreme example of refractive hyperopia. An eye with axial hyperopia has normal refractive power, but the axial length is shorter than normal. These concepts are summarized in Table 13-1.

In reality, most refractive errors have both a refractive and an axial component. Astigmatic refractive errors will be dealt with in the next chapter, but, in brief here, astigmatic eyes have two focal lines instead of a single focal point. Astigmatic refractive errors are defined by the location of the focal lines of the eye relative to the retina.

FAR POINTS AND FAR LINES

Far points and far lines are entirely different from focal points and lines. The far point (or lines) of a nonaccommodating eye is (are) determined by turning the light around, as if it were coming *from* the retina and by determining where it would come to a focus (Fig. 13-2). If the light rays emerge from the eye parallel (with zero vergence) the eye is emmetropic. If the light

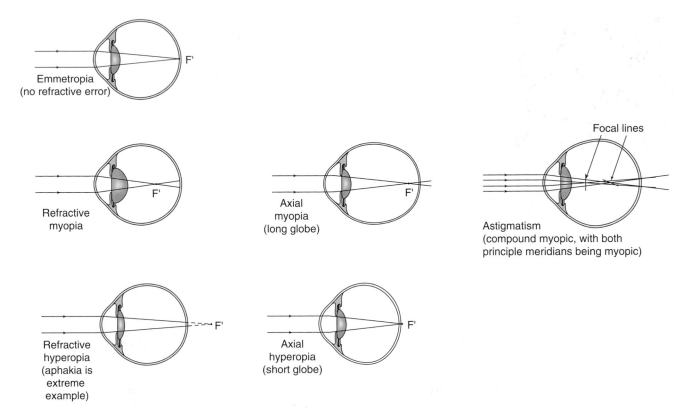

Fig. 13-1   Refractive errors are defined by the position of the secondary focal point, or focal lines, with respect to the retina, with accommodation fully relaxed. The secondary focal point of a myopic eye is the front of the retina inside the vitreous, whereas the focal point of a hyperopic eye is behind the retina.

Table 13-1   Ametropia

Ametropia	Refractive apparatus (cornea and lens) is	Axial length is
Axial myopia	Normal	Too long
Refractive myopia	Too Strong	Normal
Axial hyperopia	Normal	Too short
Refractive hyperopia	Too weak	Normal

Box 13-1   The Far Point Concept and the Correction of Ametropia

1. Locate the far point of the (nonaccommodating) eye.
2. Choose a lens with a secondary focal point that coincides with the far point of that eye.

rays are converging when they exit, the eye has a far point between the cornea and infinity, and the eye is myopic. In the hyperopic eye, the light rays are diverging when they exit, and the eye has a far point *beyond* infinity: It is a virtual far point located behind the eye. In contrast with focal points and lines (located just millimeters from the retina), far points and lines may be centimeters, meters, or even kilometers from the eye. The far point of the nonaccommodating eye is conjugate to the retina.

THE FAR POINT CONCEPT AND THE CORRECTION OF AMETROPIA

The power of a refractive correction for a given eye can be chosen by first locating the far point of that eye. An appropriate lens is chosen such that the lens' secondary focal point coincides with the far point of that eye, as shown in Fig. 13-3. The correction of ametropia using the far point concept is summarized in Box 13-1.

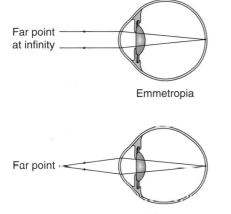

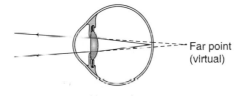

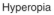

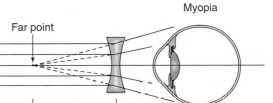

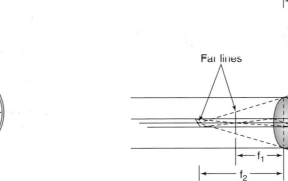

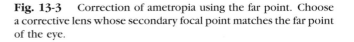

Fig. 13-2 Far points of an emmetropic, a myopic, a hyperoppic, and an astigmatic eye. Far points are determined by turning the light around, as if it were coming from the retina.

Fig. 13-3 Correction of ametropia using the far point. Choose a corrective lens whose secondary focal point matches the far point of the eye.

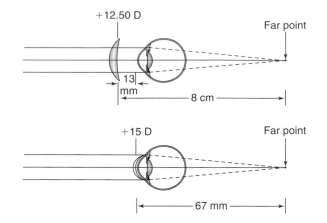

Fig. 13-5   Vertex distance in a conversion in an aphakic eye.

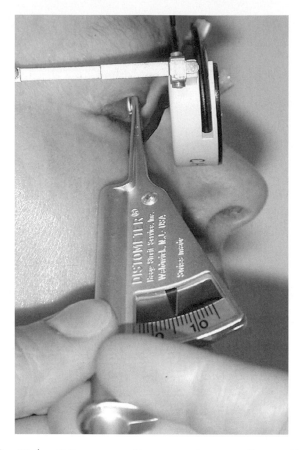

Fig. 13-4   Calipers are used to measure the vertex distance. One side contacts the posterior surface of the lens and the other the patient's closed eyelid. The reading on the scale takes into account the thickness of the lid.

Box 13-2   Vertex Distance Conversion

1. Locate the focal point of the current lens. This also locates the far point of the eye.
2. Determine the distance of the new lens to the far point of the eye. This is the focal length of the new lens.
3. Take the reciprocal of the new distance to determine the dioptric power of the new lens.

Note: Vertex distance conversion is important for powers greater than ± 5 D.

VERTEX DISTANCE

The distance between the cornea and the refractive correction is the vertex distance, sometimes abbreviated VD. The VD is zero for contact lenses and for spectacle lenses is typically between 10 and 15 mm, depending on facial anatomy, frame selection, and frame fit. As discussed in the previous section, the *position* of the re-

fractive correction can be changed, with changes made accordingly in the *power* of the refractive correction. VD conversion becomes clinically significant with refractive correction powers greater than 5 D. The method for changing the power of the refractive correction is outlined in Box 13-2.

Clinical Application—Vertex Distance Measurement and Conversion

VD can be measured in several ways. Some trial frames have rulers that allow assessment of VD. Many phoropters have prisms that also permit VD measurement, but the position of the eye relative to the phoropter can vary significantly during the refraction. The author discourages prescribing from phoropter refraction without placing the prescription in trial frames for patients where VD is an important consideration. The VD can be most accurately assessed using a caliper to measure the VD in a trial frame (Fig. 13-4).

Consider an aphakic eye that is corrected with a +12.50 D spectacle lens with a VD of 13 mm, as shown in Fig. 13-5, *top*. The focal length of the +12.50 D lens is 8 cm (0.08 m or 80 mm). This also locates the far point of the eye. Because the eye is aphakic, we know that the far point is behind the eye. If contact lens correction is desired, with a VD of 0 mm, the VD is subtracted from the focal length of the spectacle correction:

$$80 \text{ mm} - 13 \text{ mm} = 67 \text{ mm or } 0.067 \text{ m}.$$

This is the focal length of the new lens (Fig. 13-5, *bottom*), and by taking the reciprocal of the focal length to find the dioptric power of the new lens,

$$D_{\text{new lens}} = 1/0.067 \text{ m} = 15 \text{ D}.$$

Notice that with high hyperopia, the power of the contact lens is always greater than that in the spectacle plane, as discussed next. The opposite is true for eyes with myopia.

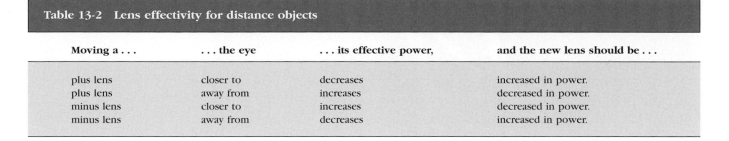

Table 13-2 Lens effectivity for distance objects			
Moving a . . .	. . . the eye	. . . its effective power,	and the new lens should be . . .
plus lens	closer to	decreases	increased in power.
plus lens	away from	increases	decreased in power.
minus lens	closer to	increases	decreased in power.
minus lens	away from	decreases	increased in power.

LENS EFFECTIVITY

Because of VD considerations, changes in the VD of the correcting lens can lead to a lens having more or less *effective* power than intended; this phenomenon is termed lens effectivity.

For distant objects (see "Suggested Readings" for a discussion of the effects at near), moving a plus lens away from the eye increases its effective plus power. A person with undercorrected hyperopia might slide his or her glasses down the nose to gain more effective plus power. In contrast, moving a plus lens closer to the eye decreases its effective power. The plus lens in the new position must be increased in power (think of it as needing to have a shorter focal length to match the far point of the eye, such as the contact lens of an aphakic eye). These concepts are summarized in Table 13-2.

Clinical Example

As discussed in the preceding section, moving a plus lens closer to the eye decreases its effective plus power, which means that the power of the new lens must be increased (Fig. 13-6). For an aphakic eye with a normal axial length and corneal curvature, an intraocular lens (IOL) of about +18.00 is required (Fig. 13-6, *bottom*). As an approximation, we can estimate that 1.25 to 1.5 D of IOL power is needed per 1.00 D of power change in the spectacle plane. Thus if 1 D myopia were desired in an eye that is calculated to need a +18.00 D IOL for emmetropia, a +19.50 D lens could be implanted. Conversely, if 1 D of hyperopia were desired, a +16.50 IOL could be implanted.

THE ERROR LENS CONCEPT

An "error lens" is a useful mathematical construct that helps to simplify optical and clinical problems, especially those involving magnification and the correction of ametropia, and when viewing an ametropic eye's fundus with a direct ophthalmoscope.

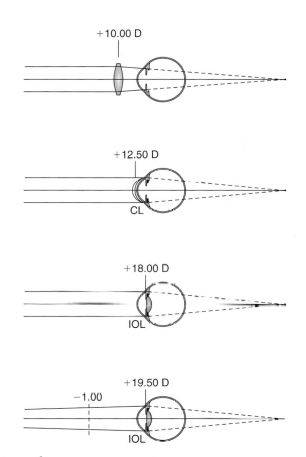

Fig. 13-6   Because of lens effectivity, the power of the refractive correction of an aphakic eye depends upon the location of the correction.

With the error lens concept, the refractive error of the eye is assumed to be entirely refractive in nature. Thus an eye with 10 D of myopia can be thought of as having a +10 D error lens. An eye with high hyperopia can accordingly be thought of as having a minus power error lens. This concept is further developed in Chapter 17 on magnification.

SUGGESTED READING

Rubin ML: The sliding lens paradox, or the unexpected effect of longitudinal ("to-and-fro") motion of plus spectacle lenses, *Surv Ophthalmol* 17(3):180-195, 1972.

Astigmatic Lenses

In previous chapters, calculations dealt with spherical lenses that had a constant radius of curvature in all meridians. This chapter will introduce and discuss cylindrical and spherocylindrical (astigmatic) lenses. Corneal and lens shape/rotation changes can cause astigmatism in the human eye and are clinically important in the examination of the eye and treatment of disease states. Retinal lesions do not cause astigmatism.

THE ASTIGMATIC LENS: PLANOCYLINDRICAL

A spherical lens can be described by the location of its focal *point;* an astigmatic (*a,* not, *stigma,* point) lens cannot. Instead, it can be described by the location of its focal *lines.* Practically speaking, an astigmatic lens has a toric surface that can be described by its maximum and minimum radii of curvature. The outside edge of a doughnut is an example of a toric surface. The powers of the two principal radii of curvature form two focal lines.

The simplest toric surface to consider is a planoconvex cylindrical lens, as shown in Fig. 14-1. This lens can be thought of as a glass cylinder cut in half lengthwise, with a finite radius of curvature around its circumference and an infinite radius of curvature along its length. (A flat surface has an infinite radius of curvature.) The effect of such a lens in an optical system depends upon the orientation in which it is held. The orientation of the lens is specified by its axis.

By convention, the notation "plano + 3.00 × 180" describes a planoconvex lens with its *axis* at 180°, but with the *power* of the lens acting in the 90° meridian. This lens has 3 D of power acting in the 90° meridian, but none acting in the 180° meridian. A focal line is formed, *parallel to the axis,* by the power acting in the 90° meridian.

THE "POWER CROSS," OR CROSS DIAGRAM: PLANOCYLINDRICAL LENS

A power cross, or cross diagram, can be constructed to represent the power of the lens acting in that meridian. This is a mathematical and geometric construct to aid understanding of the power of an astigmatic lens. It cannot be emphasized enough to the beginning student that *power crosses represent the power acting in a specified meridian!*

In Fig. 14-2, a planoconcave cylindrical lens of −4.00 × 45 is diagrammed. This planoconcave lens is oriented with its axis in the 45° meridian; its power acts in the 135° meridian. Remember that a power cross is constructed with its axes labeled with the power acting in each meridian. In this case, a −4.00 × 45 lens is represented, with 0 D of power acting in the 45° meridian and −4.00 D of power acting in the 135° meridian.

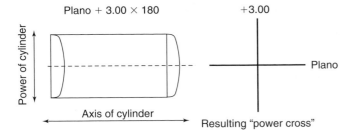

Plano + 3.00 × 180   +3.00

Axis of cylinder   Resulting "power cross"

Fig. 14-1   A planoconvex cylinder of plano + 3.00 × 180 with the resulting "power cross."

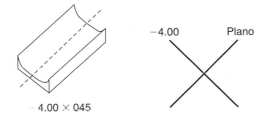

−4.00   Plano

− 4.00 × 045

Fig. 14-2   Schematic and power cross representation of a plano-concave cylindrical lens of −4.00 × 45.

THE ASTIGMATIC LENS: SPHEROCYLINDRICAL

A sphere and a cylinder may be combined to form a spherocylindrical lens, an astigmatic lens with power over the whole of its lens. This lens has two principle meridians of power acting at 90° to each other, corresponding to the maximum and minimum radii of curvature. Interestingly, a lens with identical resultant power can also be constructed by the addition of two cylinders at 90° to each other, as shown in Figure 14-3.

Great care should be taken when one converts spherocylindrical notation to power crosses and vice versa, because careless mathematical errors can occur. Remember that power crosses represent the *power* acting in a meridian, and longhand spherocylindrical notation (e.g., +4.25 + 3.50 × 70) specifies the *axis* of the cylinder.

TRANSPOSITION OF PLUS TO MINUS CYLINDER NOTATION

The power of a spherocylindrical lens can be written in minus or plus cylinder notation, and there are times when the two must be converted. The method to convert the "old" lens to the "new" lens is as follows and is summarized in Box 14-1. To determine the power of the new sphere, add the power of the old sphere to the power of the old cylinder—maintain the signs! The power of the new cylinder is the same as the power of the old cylinder, but the sign is changed. The axis of the new cylinder is obtained by changing the sign of the old cylinder by 90°, arriving at a number between 0° and 180°.

For example, +6.25 − 2.50 × 140 is transposed to plus cylinder notation as follows:

New sphere = old sphere + old cylinder

= +6.25 − 2.50 = +3.75

New cylinder = +2.50 (same power as old, with new sign)

New axis = 140 − 90 = 50°

or,

+6.25 − 2.50 × 140 ↔ +3.75 + 2.50 × 50.

SPHERICAL EQUIVALENT

The spherical equivalent of a lens is the average spherical power, in diopters, of an astigmatic lens. It is calculated by adding one-half of the cylindrical power to the spherical power of the lens:

Spherical equivalent (*D*) = sphere + ½ cylinder.

For example:

the spherical equivalent of the lens −10.00 − 2.50 × 043 is

Spherical equivalent = −10.00 + (−1.25) = −11.25 D.

COMBINATION OF ASTIGMATIC LENSES

It is at times necessary to combine spherocylindrical lenses, and when the cylindrical portions of the lenses are at the same axis or at 90° to each other, the combination is relatively straightforward. Consider the addition of the following lenses where the axis of the cylindrical correction is the same:

+8.50 + 2.25 × 90 with −0.75 + 0.50 × 90.

These can simply be added together:

+8.50 + 2.25 × 90
−0.75 + 0.50 × 90
—————————————
+7.75 + 2.75 × 90.

When the cylinders are at 90° to each other, one must first transpose the spherocylindrical notation so that the axis of the cylindrical power is the same. If +8.50 + 2.25 × 90 is to be combined with −0.75 + 0.50 × 180, one of the notations must be transposed before adding the lenses together.

Discussion continued on next page

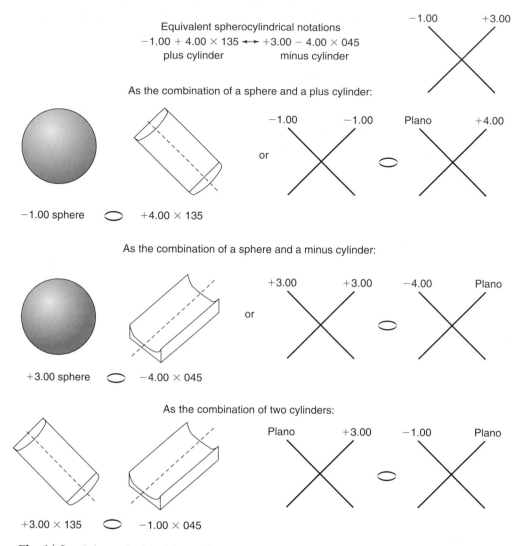

Fig. 14-3   Spherocylindrical lens. The lens may be expressed in plus or minus cylinder, and diagrammed with power crosses. Equivalent combinations are shown.

Box 14-1	Transposition of Spherocylindrical Notation

New sphere = old sphere + old cylinder
New cylinder = old cylinder, but with opposite sign
New axis = old axis changed by 90°

$$-0.75 + 0.50 \times 180 \leftrightarrow -0.25 - 0.50 \times 90$$

$$\begin{array}{r} +8.50 + 2.25 \times 90 \\ -0.25 - 0.50 \times 90 \\ \hline +8.25 + 1.75 \times 90 \end{array}$$

When the cylinders are not at the same (or at 90° away) axis, the cylinders are said to be at oblique axes. The method for combining cylinders at obliques axes follows next.

COMBINATION OF CYLINDERS AT OBLIQUE AXES

Occasionally it is necessary to combine cylinders at oblique axes, as in the overrefraction of a patient with high myopia. Historically, before the introduction of intraocular lenses (IOLs), this was a very common clinical situation in the refraction of the patient with aphakia. Even with IOLs, it is still often necessary to refract a patient with a large refractive error, and the most accurate method is to use the current glasses as a starting point and perform overrefraction with trial lens clips, as shown in Fig. 14-4. After the refraction, the patient's current prescription must be combined with the overrefraction. This can be accomplished by using one of three means: (1) using a complicated trigonometric formula, (2) using a dedicated calculator, or (3) reading the power of the combined lenses in a lensmeter.

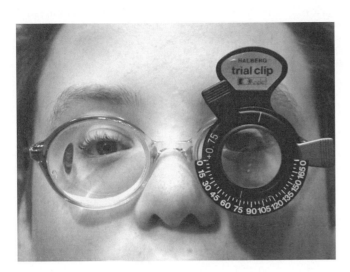

Fig. 14-4   This teen with Stickler Syndrome and high myopia is best refracted using his frames and a trial lens clip to perform an overrefraction.

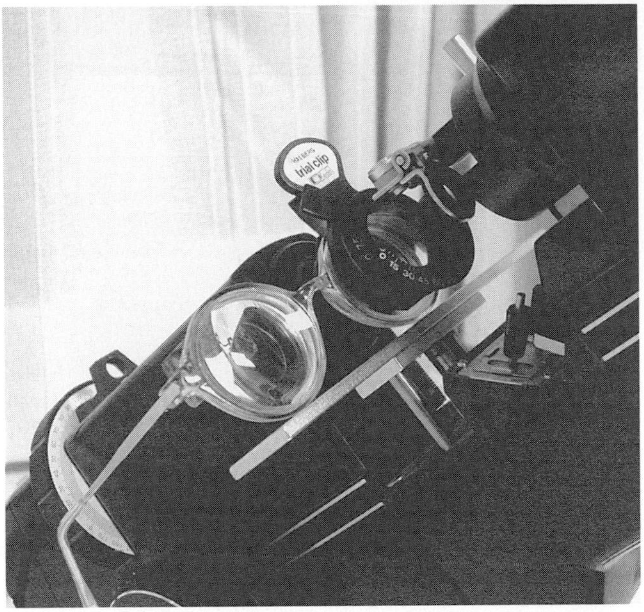

Fig. 14-5   After performing an overrefraction with trial lens clips, the combination is carefully placed in a lensmeter, where the resultant combination is read.

Most clinicians would find it cumbersome to use a trigonometric formula in the midst of a busy clinic. Dedicated calculators used to be sold for this purpose but are no longer available and would be considered bulky by today's standards. The most practical method is to read the power of the combined lenses in a lensmeter, but one must be careful not to change the axis of the cylinder when placing the glasses on the stage of the lensmeter (Fig. 14-5).

TYPES OF ASTIGMATISM

In the eye, astigmatism is caused by the cornea or the lens. Clinically, most astigmatism is corneal in origin, but the clinician must be constantly reconciling the patient's refraction and keratometry (K) readings to detect lenticular astigmatism. Retinal lesions do not cause astigmatism!

Astigmatic errors are described by the location of the secondary focal lines relative to the retina (Fig. 14-6). Compound myopic astigmatism results when both of the principle meridians are myopic, pulling the focal lines off the retina into the vitreous. In simple myopic astigmatism, one meridian is emmetropic and the other is myopic; one focal line is on the retina and the other is pulled into the vitreous. Similar definitions apply for simple and compound hyperopic astigmatism. Mixed astigmatism results when one meridian is hyperopic and the other is myopic.

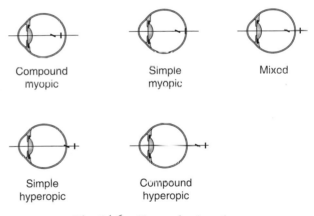

Compound myopic   Simple myopic   Mixed

Simple hyperopic   Compound hyperopic

Fig. 14-6   Types of astigmatism.

An additional way to describe astigmatism is based on the axis of the correcting cylinder. When the axis of the correcting plus cylinder is at 90° (±20°), or the axis of the correcting minus cylinder is at 180° (±20°), the astigmatism is "with-the-rule." In the absence of lenticular astigmatism, this signifies a cornea that is steeper in the vertical meridian. The correcting plus cylinder (with axis 90° [±20°], power *acting* in the 180° meridian) in effect adds more power to the 180° meridian. When the axis of the correcting plus cylinder is at 180° (±20°) or the axis of the correcting minus cylinder is at 90° (±20°), the astigmatism is "against-the-rule." In the absence of lenticular astigmatism, this signifies a cornea that is steeper in the horizontal meridian. The correcting plus cylinder (with axis 180° [±20°], power *acting* in the 90° merid-

Table 14-1   Astigmatism nomenclature

Type	Typical age	Cornea is steeper in	K readings are bigger at (±20°)	Axis of correcting plus cylinder	Axis of correcting minus cylinder (±20°)
With-the-rule	Younger	Vertical meridian	90°	90°	180°
Against-the-rule	Older	Horizontal meridian	180°	180°	90°

ian) in effect adds more power to the 90° meridian. Young people typically have with-the-rule astigmatism, and older adults have against-the-rule astigmatism (Table 14-1). (Note this clinical pearl of wisdom: Infants will often have against-the-rule astigmatism, whereas children typically have with-the-rule astigmatism.) Astigmatism is oblique when the axis of the correcting cylinder is outside the above axes.

KERATOMETRY READINGS

K readings specify the dioptric power of the cornea, although the keratometer itself really determines the curvature of the anterior corneal surface by measuring the size of a mire reflected from the central cornea. Although the measure of the radius of curvature of the anterior surface is exact, the dioptric power is calculated using the formula for the power of a refracting surface:

$$D = n - n'/r.$$

A keratometric refractive index of 1.3375 is used to take into account the minus power of the posterior surface of the cornea, so the formula becomes

$$D = 1.3375 - 1.0000/\text{measured radius of curvature}.$$

Thus a K reading of 42.00 is equivalent to a radius of curvature of 8.04 mm, and a K reading of 44.00 is equivalent of a radius of 7.67 mm, as detailed in Table 14-2.

K readings of 44.00 sphere denote a spherical cornea, whereas readings of 42.00/44.00 @ 80 represent a cornea with 42 D of power acting in the 170° meridian and 44 D acting in the 80° meridian, as shown in Fig. 14-7. This cornea is steeper (smaller radius of curvature, or more steeply curved) in the 80° meridian and flatter (larger radius of curvature) in the 170° meridian. This eye has with-the-rule astigmatism and (assuming the astigmatism is corneal) would require about +2.00 × 80 (or −2.00 × 170) correction in addition to any spherical component in the refractive correction. When calculating the axis and power of the correcting cylinder, think about making one meridian more (plus cylinder correction) or less (minus cylinder correction) powerful. Thus if the K read-

Table 14-2   K readings: radius of curvature

K	Radius (mm)
40.00	8.44
41.00	8.23
42.00	8.04
43.00	7.85
44.00	7.67
45.00	7.50
46.00	7.34
47.00	7.18
48.00	7.03
49.00	6.89
50.00	6.75

ings are known, the axis and power of the correcting cylindrical lens can be derived (and there is no lenticular astigmatism). However, the spherical power of the refractive correction cannot be calculated unless the spherical equivalent is known, as discussed next.

Consider the following example, illustrated in Fig. 14-8. An eye has K readings of 43.50/45.00 @ 90. Using spheres only, the patient reads 20/25 with −2.50 D correction. Assuming there is no lenticular astigmatism, it is known that the spherical equivalent of the correction is −2.50 D, and the power and axis of the correcting plus cylinder is +1.50 × 90 (or −1.50 × 180). Remember that

Spherical equivalent = sphere + ½ cylinder.

Rearranging,

Sphere = spherical equivalent − ½ cylinder.

In this example,

Sphere = −2.50 − 0.75 = −3.25

so the refractive correction should be

−3.25 +1.50 × 90 ↔ − 1.75 − 1.50 × 180.

Note that K readings are similar to power crosses in that they describe the power acting in that meridian.

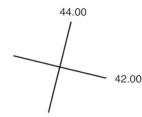
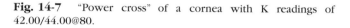

Fig. 14-7 "Power cross" of a cornea with K readings of 42.00/44.00@80.

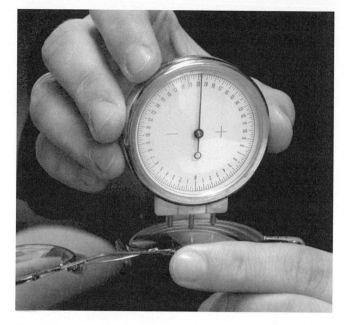

Fig. 14-9 A Geneva lens clock is used to measure the curvature of the front surface of a spectacle lens.

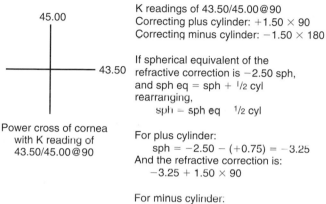

45.00

43.50

Power cross of cornea with K reading of 43.50/45.00@90

K readings of 43.50/45.00@90
Correcting plus cylinder: +1.50 × 90
Correcting minus cylinder: −1.50 × 180

If spherical equivalent of the refractive correction is −2.50 sph, and sph eq = sph + 1/2 cyl rearranging,
sph = sph eq − 1/2 cyl

For plus cylinder:
sph = −2.50 − (+0.75) = −3.25
And the refractive correction is:
−3.25 + 1.50 × 90

For minus cylinder:
sph = −2.50 − (−0.75) = −1.75
And the refractive correction is:
−1.75 − 1.50 × 180

Fig. 14-8 Calculating the prescription of an eye with K readings of 43.50/45.00@90, and a spherical equivalent of −2.50 sphere.

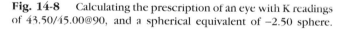

Box 14-2 Uses of the Geneva Lens Clock

Determine whether a lens has a toric surface.
Identify a warped lens.
Compare the base curves of two lenses if a patient is dissatisfied with new glasses.

CLINICAL APPLICATION: WHICH STITCH TO CUT OR WHERE IS THE GAPE?

K readings can be used to help a surgeon decide which stitch(es) is (are) too tight or too loose after surgery (e.g., surgery for penetrating ocular trauma, cataract surgery with larger wounds, or penetrating keratoplasty), especially if the preoperative K readings are known. Tight sutures near the limbus cause peripheral flattening—at the expense of central corneal steepening—in the axis of the tight suture. Wound gape usually causes flattening of the K readings in that axis.

For instance, if a patient had K readings of 44.50 sphere before cataract surgery with a superior limbal incision, and postoperatively had K readings of 42.00/46.00 @ 87, a tight suture (or two!) near the 12 o'clock position might be expected. Similarly, flat K readings can point to wound gape or to limbal melt caused by connective tissue disorders.

LENS GAUGE (GENEVA LENS CLOCK)

A lens gauge (Fig. 14-9) measures the radius of curvature of a lens and can determine the dioptric power of a surface if the index of refraction of the material is known (much like a keratometer). An individual lens gauge is calibrated for use with a specific material with a specified index of refraction. The lens gauge has three prongs at its base; the outer two are fixed and the middle prong is movable. The direction and amount of displacement of the central prong relative to the two outer prongs determine whether the surface is concave, flat, or convex and its radius of curvature. A Geneva lens clock made for use on crown glass lenses can be used on a plastic lens to read the radius of curvature, but the scale for dioptric power should be disregarded. One must be careful not to scratch the plastic lens with the prongs! The uses of a Geneva lens clock are summarized in Box 14-2.

THE CONOID OF STURM

Understanding the concept of the conoid of Sturm often strikes fear in the hearts of beginning ophthalmic optics students. It is simply the name of the geometric figure that is formed by a pencil of light rays refracted by a circular spherocylindrical lens. The easiest case to consider is parallel light incident upon a spherocylindrical lens that has plus power in both of its meridians. A pencil of light with zero vergence that is refracted by a spherocylindrical lens will form two focal lines. The focal line closer to the lens will be formed by the power acting in the dioptrically more powerful meridian, and a second focal line will be formed further from the lens by the less powerful meridian. The geometric figure formed by the solid shape between the two focal lines is called the conoid of Sturm, as shown in Fig. 14-10. (In the case of parallel incident light and a lens that has plus power in both meridians, it can be thought of as the cardboard cylinder from a roll of paper towels that is pinched at both ends 90° to one another.) The interval of Sturm is the distance between the two lines. The shape of the figure between the two lines varies in a characteristic manner, changing from a line, to an oval, to a circle, to an oval (90° to the first oval), to a line (90° to the first line). At one point along the optical axis, the cross section of the conoid is circular, and this corresponds to the circle of least confusion, which lies dioptrically half way in between the two focal lines and is located by the focal length of the spherical equivalent of the spherocylindrical lens.

Clinical Example

The conoid of Sturm can be demonstrated with a simple optical setup. Use a bright flashlight as a point source in a dark room. At least 1 m to the right of the source, hold in one hand a +6.00 sphere and a +4.00 cylinder × 90. Use the other hand to gradually move a piece of paper away from the lenses. At first there will be a vertically oriented oval, and then there will be a vertically oriented line that corresponds to the focal line formed by the combination of the +6.00 sphere and the +4.00 cylinder × 90: +10 D of power acting in the 180° meridian. The cross section will become vertically oval again and next forms a circle. The circle corresponds to the circle of least confusion and is formed by the spherical equiv-

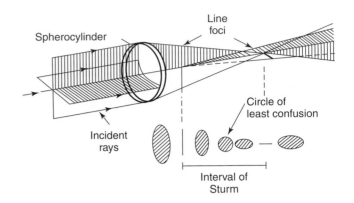

Fig. 14-10   Conoid of Sturm.

alent of the lens (+8.00 D). After the circle of least confusion, the cross section becomes horizontally oval and then becomes a horizontally oriented line, corresponding to the focal line formed by the +6.00 D acting in the 90° meridian, but with its axis at 180°. After the more distant focal line, the cross section once again becomes horizontally oval. The order, location, and orientation of the focal lines depend upon the vergence of the light rays entering the lens and the power of the astigmatic lens; a "conoid" is formed as long as the aperture is circular.

Clinical Application: Refraction Using the Astigmatic Dial

Certain methods of refraction (e.g., use of the astigmatic dial, *not* cross-cylinder subjective refraction) are based upon moving first one secondary focal line onto the retina and then collapsing the conoid of Sturm onto the retina with cylindrical lenses. Both focal lines are brought into the eye (in front of the retina) by fogging the eye with plus sphere. Next, minus sphere is added until the patient reports that one line of the astigmatic dial appears blackest and sharpest. The axis of the correcting minus cylinder is oriented perpendicular to that line. Minus cylinder power is added until all lines are equally black and sharp; this collapses the more anterior focal line of the conoid of Sturm onto the retina.

SUGGESTED READING

Rubin ML: *Optics for Clinicians,* ed 3, Gainesville, Fla., 1977, Triad.

Prisms

Prisms are widely used in ophthalmology in the assessment of acuity and sensory function, the measurement of strabismus and motility disorders, and the treatment of diplopia. Moderate amounts of base-up or base-down prism can be used to evaluate the fixation preference of infants and preliterate/nonverbal patients without gross ocular misalignment. Small amounts of base out prism (e.g., the 4Δ base-out test) can be useful in the evaluation of suppression. Prisms are essential in the accurate measurement and diagnosis of strabismic deviations and for planning surgical intervention. They are also used to measure vergence amplitudes of patients with potential disorders of convergence and divergence, as well as vertical fusional amplitudes in the patients with possible fourth nerve palsies. Prisms are used therapeutically for patients with diplopia, vergence disorders, anomalous head positions, or visual field limitations and can be used cosmetically in patients with disfigurement. A prism is used as ballast to properly orient the cylinder axis in toric contact lenses. Finally, prisms are a common component of ophthalmic instruments. A thorough knowledge of prisms is desirable in all areas of ophthalmic practice.

WHAT IS A PRISM?

A prism is a wedge of refracting material with non-parallel faces and a triangular cross-section with an apex and a base (Fig. 15-1). Prisms may be either isosceles or right angle in cross-section. Light is refracted at each surface as it enters and exits the prism; the total angle of deviation is the sum of the deviations produced at each of the faces. Although the *total* deviation is always in the direction of the base of the prism, the two deviations may be in the same or opposite direction, depending on the angle of incidence of the entering light (Fig. 15-2). The minimum angle of deviation occurs when the angles of deviation produced at the two faces are equal, as seen in Fig. 15-2, *A*. The angle of deviation in any other position is always greater. The Prentice position occurs when the incident ray is perpendicular to the surface.

IMAGE DISPLACEMENT BY PRISMS

Although the rays are bent toward the base of the prism, the image is perceived as being displaced toward the apex of the prism. Demonstrate this by using a laser pointer and a prism. Activate the laser and introduce a prism; the light will be bent toward the base of the prism. In contrast, view a target across the room and then introduce a prism; the image of the target will be seen as being displaced upward (Fig. 15-3).

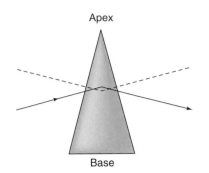

Fig. 15-1   Cross section of a prism.

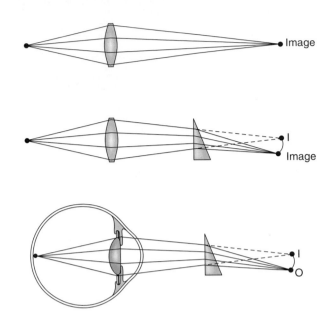

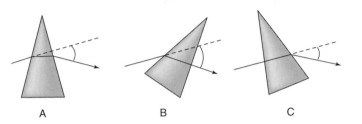

Fig. 15-2   The total deviation is always in the direction of the base of the prism, and the total deviation is the sum of the deviations produced at each face. The minimum angle of deviation is shown in *A*.

Fig. 15-3   *Top*, an image is formed by a lens. *Middle*, a prism is introduced and the image is displaced toward the base of the prism. *Bottom*, when viewing with an eye, the virtual image is seen as displaced toward the apex of the prism.

DEFINITION OF A PRISM DIOPTER

In ophthalmology the power of a prism is usually quantified in prism diopters (Δ). Each prism diopter produces 1 cm of deviation of a light ray from where it would have otherwise traveled, measured 100 cm from the prism (Fig. 15-4). Thus a 15Δ prism produces 15 cm of deviation of a light ray when measured 1 m from the prism. The same prism would produce 7.5 cm of deviation measured 50 cm from the prism and 30 cm of deviation measured 200 cm from the prism. It is important not to confuse prism diopters (Δ) with diopters (D) or with degrees, for the meanings are quite different.

Although the total angle of deviation of a light ray by a prism is a trigonometric function [degrees = $\tan^{-1}(\Delta/100)$], some clinically useful approximations can be made. For angles less than 45° (equal to 100Δ), each 2Δ of angular deviation is *approximately* equal to 1° (actually closer to 1.7Δ per degree). For angles greater than 45°, this approximation is not correct, because each degree of angular deviation eventually approaches an infinite number of prism diopters.

CALIBRATION OF PRISMS

Because the total deviation of a light ray by a prism can vary depending on the angle of incidence of the entering

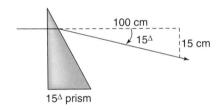

Fig. 15-4   A prism diopter produces 1 cm of deviation from where it would have otherwise traveled; measured 100 cm from the prism. A 15$^\Delta$ prism is illustrated.

ray (see Fig. 15-2), it is important to hold the prism in the position specified by the manufacturer to obtain the power marked on the prism. Although the errors introduced by improper prism positioning (Prentice position versus frontal plane position and vice versa) are relatively small with lower prism powers, they can become clinically significant with higher prism powers and grossly incorrect prism positioning. Measurement errors lead to inaccurate surgical dosing for strabismus surgery and undesirable surgical outcomes. A prism is labeled with a power that is accurate when it is held in the position specified by the manufacturer.

Older orthoptic prisms made from glass are generally calibrated to be held in the Prentice position (Fig. 15-5, *B*), with the rear surface of the prism held perpendicular to the line of sight of the deviated eye. Prism in spectacle lenses is also measured in the Prentice position with the rear face of the corrective lens perpendicular to the

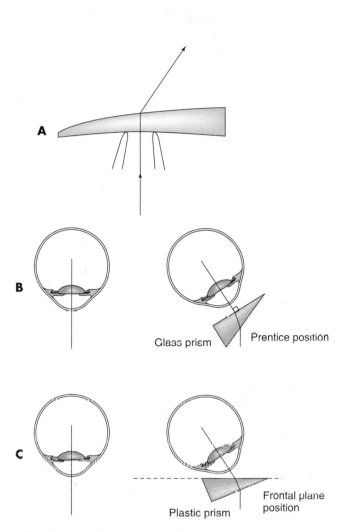

Fig. 15-5   A, Prism in spectacle lenses is measured in the Prentice position, with the rear face of the prism perpendicular to the nosecone of the lensmeter. **B,** Older glass prisms are calibrated to be held in the Prentice position. **C,** Plastic prisms are calibrated to be held in the angle of minimum deviation, which turns out to be very close to frontal plane position. The rear face of the prism is held perpendicular to the frontal plane of the individual.

nosecone of the lensmeter. In contrast, most modern plastic orthoptic prisms and prism bars are calibrated to be held in the angle of minimum deviation. This turns out to be quite close to the frontal plane position, and the measurement errors introduced by the positioning difference (frontal plane position instead of angle of minimum deviation) are slight and clinically insignificant.

Clinical Use of Prisms in Evaluation of Ocular Motility

When one measures ocular alignment outside of the primary position, it is important to maintain proper positioning of the prisms as discussed in the preceding sec-

tion. In upgaze and downgaze, the prism should be held with the rear face perpendicular to the floor and in the frontal plane position. Vertical and horizontal orientation of the prisms relative to the face and eyes should be maintained with head tilt right and left. In right-gaze and left-gaze, the prism is held in the frontal plane position in front of the nonfixating eye.

Orthoptic prisms are available in powers up to 50Δ, but larger angles of strabismus should be measured by holding prisms in front of both eyes instead of "stacking." Prisms should *never* be stacked in the same direction (i.e., two base-out prisms in front of the same eye to measure a large-angle esotropia) because the second prism is not being held in its properly calibrated position. For deviations greater than 50Δ, a second prism should be held in front of the fellow eye, and the total resultant deviation read from a table (see Thompson and Guyton, "Suggested Reading" at the end of this chapter). In contrast, a combined horizontal and vertical deviation can be measured with the prisms stacked together without introducing measurement errors.

In patients with paralytic or restrictive strabismus, it is essential to specify the eye with which the patient is fixating. In paralytic strabismus, the deviation measured when the patient is fixating with the paretic eye ("secondary" deviation) will be larger than that measured with the nonparetic eye fixating ("primary" deviation) because of Hering's law. Serial measurements recorded without specifying the fixating eye can lead to a false impression of improvement or worsening of a patient's condition, potentially leading to inappropriate management that is expensive or dangerous. Similarly, patients with restrictive strabismus (e.g., Brown's syndrome or strabismus caused by secondary to thyroid eye disease) may appear to have a different deviation depending upon which eye is fixing.

PRISMATIC EFFECT OF LENSES— PRENTICE'S RULE

At the optical center of a lens, there is no prismatic power. A ray passing through the optical center of a lens passes through the lens undeviated. A ray that passes through the lens away from the optical center is bent toward the optical center in plus lenses (Fig. 15-6) and away from the optical center in minus lenses. The amount of deviation depends on the power of the lens and the distance away from the optical center and is described by Prentice's rule:

$$\Delta \text{ (prism diopters)} = h \text{ (cm from the center)} \times D \text{ (dioptric power of the lens)}.$$

Prentice's rule and the prismatic effect of lenses become clinically important when one is purposefully de-

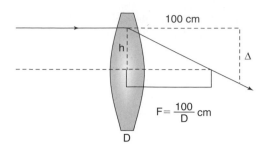

Fig. 15-6   A ray that passes through a plus lens away from its optical center is bent toward the optical center, and the amount is calculated using Prentice's rule (see text).

Box 15-1   Methods to Incorporate Prism into Refractive Correction

Grond-in prism
Decentration of lens(es)
Fresnel Press-on prism
Bicentric grinding
Edge-to-edge bonding

---

centering lenses to induce prism, as well as in patients with anisometropic spectacle correction in the reading position. Prismatic effects of bifocal lenses must also be taken into account when one is prescribing reading adds to minimize image jump and image displacement.

INCORPORATING PRISMS INTO SPECTACLE CORRECTION

There are several ways prisms can be prescribed and dispensed in a patient's prescription (Box 15-1). Prisms may be purposefully incorporated into glasses when the lenses are made at the optical shop or added to the glasses later with a Fresnel Press-on prism. A prism can be permanently added by decentering a higher power spectacle lens according to Prentice's rule or by grinding the prism into the lens using shims in the lens lathe. Aspheric and progressive addition lenses are not suitable for decentration, and the prism must be ground onto the back of the lens. Fresnel Press-on prisms are useful because of their low cost and the ability to change the amount of prism if the angle of deviation is changing, as in patients with thyroid eye disease or a resolving, vasculopathic sixth nerve palsy. By using bicentric grinding, the power of a prism in the top and bottom of a lens can be different, also known as slab-off or reverse slab. Edge-to-edge bonding is another technique opticians can use to put different amounts of prism in the upper and lower portions of lenses. The top portion of the lens is ground with the specified prism, truncated, and joined to a second lens with a different amount of prism that has also been truncated. The combined lens is then finished to fit in the patient's frames. The resulting lenses look similar to Franklin-style bifocal lenses, although there may or may not be a presbyopic addition for near vision.

MEASURING PRISM IN GLASSES

To measure the prism in a patient's glasses, the point through which the patient is looking must be marked with a water-soluble, felt-tipped pen. This is very important, because the glasses may be out of alignment, inadvertently inducing prism or changing the amount of effective prism power of the glasses. The marked portion of the lens is placed on the stage of the lensmeter and the amount of prism is read according to the manufacturer's directions. Remember to note not only the amount, but also the orientation, of the prism.

PRESCRIBING AND DISPENSING PRISMS

When one prescribes a prism for incorporation into (ground-in, decentered, or bicentric grinding) or application to (Fresnel prism) a patient's glasses, it is necessary to exactly specify the amount (in prism diopters), orientation (base-in, base-out, or angle of orientation of oblique prism), and eye(s) to which the prism should be applied. Even when prismatic prescriptions are fastidiously written, unintentional prism-dispensing errors by the optical shop are common. If a patient calls with complaints after receiving a prism in the glasses, it is advisable to have the patient return to the office to make sure that the prism was properly dispensed.

When only small amounts (1 or 2Δ) of prismatic correction are needed, the prism can be put in just one spectacle lens to minimize cost to the patient. When vertical prism is necessary, consider prescribing slightly more base-up prism on one side to minimize lower edge thickness on the contralateral eye, rather than dividing the prism equally between the eyes. Horizontal prism is often split equally, except when one eye has noticeably poorer visual function, in which case relatively more prism should be placed before the poorly seeing eye. This lessens the chromatic aberration perceived by the better eye.

If both vertical and horizontal prisms are required, prescribe the prism at an oblique orientation to decrease weight and cost. Consider a patient who requires 7Δ base-out and 7Δ base-down for the right eye to alleviate diplopia. Prism could be prescribed as 7Δ base-out for the right eye (OD) and 7Δ base-up for the left eye (OS).

The same result could be achieved optically by prescribing 5Δ base-down and base-out, apex to 45° OD, and 5Δ base-out and base-up to 45° OS. The edges of the lenses would be thinner and the weight less.

Small amounts of base-down vertical prism (less than 3 or 4Δ) can be incorporated into contact lenses if needed. Horizontal prism cannot be used in contact lenses, because gravity will rotate the base of the prism inferiorly.

Slab-off, or bicentric grinding, can be used to alleviate diplopia in the reading position caused by heterophorias secondary to anisometropic corrections or to compensate for vertical strabismus that is vertically incomitant and is discussed later in this chapter.

Prisms for Diplopia

Prisms are most often prescribed by the ophthalmologist to alleviate diplopia by compensating for a strabismic deviation. Most optical laboratories can incorporate up to 10 or 12Δ into the spectacle lens of a properly selected frame, but the amount depends upon the skill of the optician and the patient's refractive correction. It is important to specify the amount of the prism, the lens(es), and the direction of the base of the prism, as discussed in the following sections.

Using Fresnel Press-on Prisms

Fresnel Press-on prisms have many uses in adult and pediatric ophthalmic practice. Their utility in identifying the proper angle for children with acquired esotropia was demonstrated in the Prism Adaptation Trial. Serial applications are usually necessary until the maximum deviation is identified. In adult patients with strabismus, Fresnel Press-on prisms are especially useful in the treatment of evolving (e.g., thyroid strabismus) or temporary (e.g., microvascular abducens palsy) ocular misalignment. Remember that visual acuity is decreased because of chromatic aberration and glare and that lenses with Fresnel prisms are difficult to keep clean.

Prisms for Head Turns

Prisms may also be prescribed to alleviate small head turns caused by nystagmus or strabismus. In the author's experience, however, a prism is seldom useful for face turns because the amount of prism necessary to alleviate significant face turn is too large to be technically or cosmetically feasible. For example, a 20° face turn to the patient's right would require

$$20° \times 1.7Δ/° = 34Δ$$

of prism in each lens, with the base at 180°. Such spectacle lenses would be unsightly and technically difficult to make. Nevertheless, prisms (permanent or Fresnel

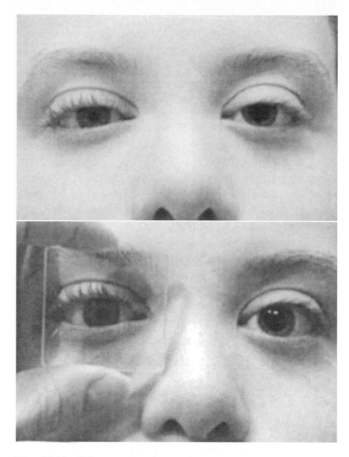

Fig. 15-7 Prism used to change the apparent location of a prosthetic right eye. Base-down prism is placed before the right eye to raise the image of that eye to the observer.

Press-on) can be used, with variable results and success, for patients with anomalous head positions associated with nystagmus or strabismus.

Prisms for Cosmesis

Prisms may be incorporated into spectacle correction to improve the cosmesis of a blind or disfigured eye or prosthesis. According to American Academy of Ophthalmology guidelines, monocular patients should wear spectacle correction on a full-time basis to protect their good eye, and thoughtful prism prescription can improve the appearance of a poorly seeing or nonseeing eye. For example, base-down prism can make a hypotropic prosthesis appear higher to the observer (Fig. 15-7).

Prisms for Visual Field Loss

Special-order lenses with multiple prisms incorporated are also available for patients with severe peripheral field constriction (e.g., retinitis pigmentosa or glaucoma) or visual field loss because of pathology in the visual pathways posterior to the chiasm. Most practitioners who treat patients with low vision report limited success with this type of lens, but do find them occasionally useful.

INDUCED PRISM IN ANISOMETROPIA

If a patient reads below the optical centers of their spectacle correction, prism is induced according to Prentice's rule (discussed earlier in this chapter). For instance, a patient wearing OD −3.00 + 1.00 × 90 and OS −0.50 + 1.50 × 180 who reads 1 cm below the optical center of the spectacle correction will experience 4Δ base-down OD (or 4Δ base-up OS) of effective prism in that position. In this example, the 4 D of anisometropia in the reading position will produce a right hypotropia.

Many patients learn to fuse small vertical deviations caused by anisometropic spectacle correction in downgaze, but there are several techniques available to deal with the diplopia in patients who do not or cannot adapt, as outlined in Box 15-2. These techniques attempt to limit or reduce the induced prismatic effects of the anisometropic correction in downgaze. Remember that it is the anisometropic correction that causes the deviation, *not* the reading add.

Patients can wear contact lenses instead of spectacle correction or can consider refractive surgery to lessen the anisometropia. The optical centers of the lenses can be lowered to compromise the vertical imbalance between distance and near. Dissimilar segments with different amounts of image displacement (not image jump) can also be used in the patient with presbyopia. A Fresnel Press-on prism can be used on the lower segment of one

---

Box 15-2   Techniques for Treating Diplopia in Downgaze Caused by Anisometropic Spectacle Correction

Contact lenses instead of spectacles
Refractive surgery to eliminate anisometropia
Lowering of both optical centers to compromise the vertical imbalance between distance and near
Separate, single-vision glasses for distance and near
Dissimilar segments if the patient is presbyopic
Fresnel Press-on prism over part of lens
Occlusion of lower half of one lens
Slab-off (bicentric) grinding

---

lens in any patient with anisometropia who has diplopia in downgaze.

Bicentric grinding can also be used to treat patients with anisometropia that leads to a vertical anisophoria and diplopia in downgaze. Because it is the anisometropic spectacle correction that causes the diplopia (not a near addition), bicentric grinding can be used for patients with misalignment that is vertically incomitant with or without a presbyopic correction.

SUGGESTED READINGS

Brooks CW, Borish IM: *System for ophthalmic dispensing,* ed 2, Boston, 1996, Butterworth-Heinemenn.
Thompson JT, Guyton DL: Ophthalmic prisms: measurement errors and how to minimize them, *Ophthalmology* 90:204-210, 1983.

Accommodation, Presbyopia, and Bifocals

Accommodative problems are some of the most common reasons that patients seek eye care. Although accommodative amplitudes are large in childhood, progressive loss of accommodative amplitude in the fourth and fifth decades leads to symptoms of presbyopia. In addition, other disease states (e.g., injuries, chronic illness, and pseudophakia) or medications can also cause these symptoms. A thorough understanding of accommodation, its loss, and the treatment of presbyopia will improve the care that a physician provides for patients with accommodative insufficiency.

ACCOMMODATION

Definitions

Accommodation is the increased convexity of the natural crystalline lens. The increased convexity adds plus power to the optical system of the eye, "pulling" the far point of the eye closer to the front of the eye. Although accommodation occurs inside the eye, it is often thought of as occurring at the cornea for purposes of calculation. *Amplitude of accommodation* is measured in diopters and is the total amount of plus power that can be effected with the accommodative mechanism.

The *far point* is the location along the line of sight that is conjugate to the retina with accommodation fully re-

laxed. An emmetrope has a far point at infinity, whereas a myope's far point is located somewhere between infinity and the front of the eye. A hyperope has a virtual far point, located behind the eye. The near point is the location on the line of sight that is conjugate to the retina with accommodation maximally active. The *range of accommodation* is the interval of clear vision obtainable along the line of sight with accommodative effort. Far point and near point are reported in centimeters or meters from the cornea.

Accommodative Norms

Classic tables published by Donders (Table 16-1) established norms for age, but it is important to recognize that there is considerable, and clinically important, individual variation. As a general rule, most people are comfortable using only half of their total accommodative amplitude on a sustained basis. In addition, refractive error and the method of correction, ambient lighting, body habitus, and task requirements must also be considered. For example, a particularly tall person will have a longer working distance than a smaller person. A person who works in bright light (e.g., a surveyor) may have smaller pupils and thus greater depth of field and fewer symptoms of presbyopia than someone who works in dimly lit situations (e.g., a waitperson in a bar).

Measurement of Accommodation

Accommodation must be measured with the proper refractive correction for distance in place and before the instillation of mydriatic and cycloplegic agents. Accommodative amplitudes are generally measured monocularly and then binocularly; the binocular amplitude of accommodation typically exceeds the monocular amplitude of accommodation by 0.5 to 1 D. Three basic methods exist to *measure* accommodative amplitude: the near point of accommodation, an accommodative rule, and the method of spheres (Box 16-1). Accommodative facility can also be evaluated with dynamic retinoscopy. It must be remembered that the measurement of accommodation requires patient cooperation.

When the near point of accommodation method is used, the patient has refractive correction for distance in place and views a near target (small print). The near target is brought toward the patient until the print blurs, and then the distance from the eye is recorded. The reciprocal of the distance (in meters) is the amplitude of accommodation in diopters. This method is useful for patients with larger amplitudes of accommodation (>3 D) and requires that accurate refractive correction for distance be in place. A word of caution: Accommodative amplitude measured with this technique will be incorrect if the patient is not wearing his or her proper distance refraction.

An accommodative rule (such as a Prince or RAF rule) can also be used to measure accommodative amplitude. Once again, the proper refractive correction for distance must be in place. A +3.00 D lens placed in front of an emmetropic (or properly corrected ametropic) eye should bring the far point in from infinity to 33 cm from the eye, where a near target should be in focus. (If the person does not begin to see the target clearly at 33 cm, the distance refractive correction is incorrect.) The near target is then brought toward the eye until the patient can no longer keep the target in focus, and the distance is recorded and converted to diopters. If a +3.00 D lens has been used, the 3 D must be subtracted from the total. For example, if a patient wearing his or her spectacles for distance vision correction sees the near target clearly from 33 to 10 cm from the eye, the accommodative amplitude would be 10 D − 3 D = 7 D.

In the gradient method, the patient has proper refractive correction for distance in place and is asked to fixate on a near target at 40 cm. Accommodation is stimulated by adding minus sphere until the print blurs, and the dioptric power required to blur the print is noted. Accommodation is then relaxed by adding plus sphere until the print blurs, which should be +2.50 D if the distance refraction is correct. The sum of the two lenses is the accommodative amplitude. For example, if the patient reports blur at −4.50 sphere and vision is clear until +2.50 sphere, the accommodative amplitude is 2.50 + 4.50 = 7 D.

When an ametrope with uncorrected presbyopia is asked to view a near target, the near point will depend upon the degree and type of ametropia and the accommodative amplitude. This is illustrated in Table 16-2. Thus, a person with uncorrected hyperopia will have a remote near point in contrast to a person with uncorrected myopia with the same degree of ametropia and accommodative amplitude. The near and far points of an ametrope with proper refractive correction will match those of an emmetrope with the same amplitude of accommodation.

Table 16-1 Accommodation and age (after Donders)

Age (years)	Accommodation (D)
1	18
5	16
10	14
15	12
20	10
25	8.5
30	7
35	5.5
40	4.5
45	4.5
50	3.5
55	1.75
60	1.00
65	0.75
70	0.25
75	0.00

Box 16-1 Methods to Measure Accommodation

Near point of accommodation
Accommodative rule
Method of spheres

Table 16-2 Effect of uncorrected ametropia on accommodative parameters

Refractive state	Amplitude of accommodation	Far point	Near point	Range of accommodation
Emmetropia	5 D	At ∞	20 cm	∞ to 20 cm
3 D Myopia	5 D	33 cm in front of eye	12.5 cm	33 to 12.5 cm
3 D Hyperopia	5 D	33 cm behind eye	50 cm	∞ to 50 cm

ACCOMMODATIVE LOSS (PRESBYOPIA)

Presbyopia is the loss of accommodative ability, which generally becomes apparent in the first half of the fifth decade. Presbyopia is most likely multifactorial, but loss of lens elasticity with age may be the most important contributing factor. Other processes may also lead to premature loss of accommodation, "accommodative insufficiency," and are listed in Box 16-2.

REFRACTIVE CORRECTION FOR ACCOMMODATIVE DEFICIENCY

To compensate for the loss of accommodation, it is necessary for the physician to prescribe lenses to aid the person to perform near tasks. The major classes of multifocal lenses are bifocals, trifocals, quadrifocals, and progressive addition lenses (Fig. 16-1). Monovision is another alternative for individuals with presbyopia and is discussed next.

Bifocals today are manufactured in Franklin style, flat top, and round top segments. Trifocals are similar to the flat top style of bifocals, with the addition of an intermediate segment at the top of the D-segment. Quadrifocals are similar to trifocals, with the addition of a segment placed above the distance segment; these are useful for patients with presbyopia who do a lot of overhead work, e.g., pilots, plumbers, or stock clerks.

Progressive Addition Lenses

Progressive addition lenses are made by grinding a plus lens onto the front of a lens with an increasing plus power toward the bottom of the lens. Although this technology affords the patient variable focus and simulates restoration of natural accommodation, it comes at the expense of peripheral irregular astigmatism. The optical aberrations caused by the peripheral lens surface can cause a swimming sensation with head movement. Small amounts of misalignment of the lenses relative to the pupils can lead to poor acuity, so proper fitting and maintenance of proper frame alignment are essential.

IMAGE JUMP AND IMAGE DISPLACEMENT

Image jump occurs with the sudden introduction of prism power as the eye encounters the top of the bifocal segment (Fig. 16-2). Because the optical center of a

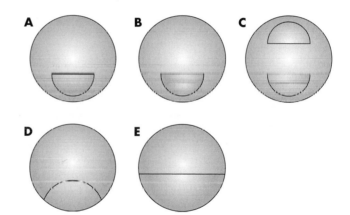

Fig. 16-1 Types of multifocal spectacle lenses: **A,** Flat-top bifocal. **B,** Trifocal. **C,** Quadrifocal. **D,** Round-top. **E,** Franklin style.

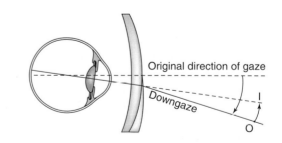

Fig. 16-2 Image jump occurs as the eye looks downward and encounters the top of the segment. If the optical center of the lens is close to the top of the segment, little (D segment) or no (Franklin) image jump occurs. If the optical center of the bifocal segment is away from the edge of the segment (round top), maximal image jump occurs. There is no image jump with progressive addition lenses.

Box 16-2 Causes of Diminished Accommodation	
PRESBYOPIA	**SYSTEMIC ILLNESS**
Aphakia/pseudophakia	Hypothyroidism
	Anemia
MEDICATIONS	Myasthenia
Phenothiazines	Diabetes
Tranquilizers	
Chloroquine	**THIRD NERVE PARESIS**
Parasympatholytics	**CILIARY GANGLION DAMAGE**
CENTRAL NERVOUS SYSTEM DISEASE	Orbital trauma
	Postsurgical
Trauma	Tonic pupil
Postencephalitis or meningitis	**CILIARY BODY DAMAGE**
	Blunt trauma
	Postsurgical
	Tumors

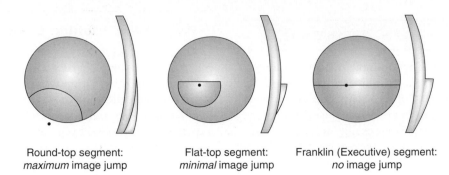

Round-top segment:
maximum image jump

Flat-top segment:
minimal image jump

Franklin (Executive) segment:
no image jump

Fig. 16-3   The effect of different types of bifocal segments on image jump.

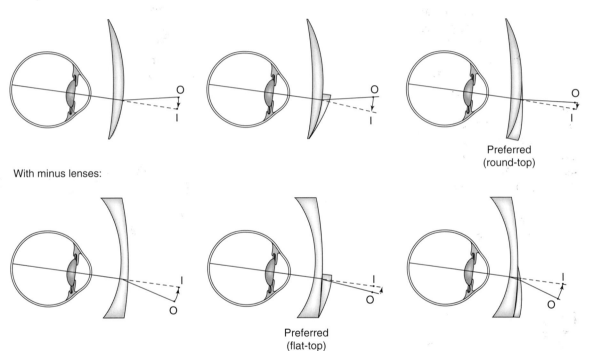

With plus lenses:

Preferred
(round-top)

With minus lenses:

Preferred
(flat-top)

Fig. 16-4   Preferred near segments have prismatic effects opposite to that of the distance segment. Thus, for plus distance lenses (prism base up), round-top near segments (prism base down) are preferred. For minus distance lenses (prism base down), flat-top near segments (prism base up) are preferred.

Franklin lens is at the top of the segment, no image jump occurs with a Franklin segment, regardless of whether the distance segment is myopic, hyperopic, or astigmatic. With a round top segment, the optical center of the add is toward the bottom of the segment, and image jump is maximal for both hyperopes and myopes. The optical center of a flat top lens is close to the top of the segment, so there is little image jump with this lens. No image jump is seen with Franklin-style lenses (Fig. 16-3).

Image displacement is the displacement produced by the total prismatic power of the distance and near segments in the reading position. Image displacement can

be minimized by choosing an add style with a prismatic effect opposite to that of the bifocal. Thus, a myope would have maximal image displacement while wearing a round top segment and minimal image displacement with a Franklin style segment (Fig. 16-4).

The effects of segment choice on image jump and displacement are summarized in Table 16-3. For a myope, it becomes obvious that the practitioner can minimize both image jump and displacement by choosing a Franklin style segment. Another choice is a flat-top segment, which performs almost as well. In contrast, the myope who wears a round top segment will have maximal image

Table 16-3	Segment choice and effect on image jump/displacement		
Distance refractive correction	Segment type	Image jump	Image displacement
Myopic	Franklin	None	Minimal
	Flat top	Almost none	Almost minimal
	Round top	Maximal	Maximal
Hyperopic	Franklin	None	Maximal
	Flat top	Almost none	Almost maximal
	Round top	Maximal	Minimal

jump and displacement. Round top segments are a poor choice for patients with myopia.

The choice is not as clear for hyperopes with presbyopia, who must choose between maximal image jump and minimal image displacement with round top segments or minimal image jump and image maximal displacement with Franklin segments. The choice of segment type thus depends upon whether the hyperope finds image jump or displacement more bothersome.

MONOVISION

Monovision describes the relative refractive state of the individual when one eye is in focus for near tasks and the fellow eye is in focus for distance. Occasional individuals have "natural" monovision, but in most cases it is an iatrogenic event. Monovision can occur as a carefully planned outcome or as an unanticipated result of cataract or refractive surgery. Monovision is a popular choice for contact lens wearers with presbyopia.

Monovision is acceptable to about 75% of the population, and, conversely, unacceptable to 25% of individuals. It is essential that those persons who will not tolerate monovision be identified before one performs surgical procedures. In refractive surgery, monovision can be evaluated before the procedure with contact lenses to make sure that monovision is acceptable to the individual.

Monovision can reduce or eliminate the individual's dependence on glasses but decreases binocularity and contrast sensitivity. It may be contraindicated in persons with amblyopia, those with manifest or latent strabismus, or those who require fine stereopsis and acute contrast sensitivity.

SUGGESTED READINGS

Jain S, Arora I, Azar DT: Success of monovision in presbyopes: review of the literature and potential applications to refractive surgery, *Surv Ophthalmol* 40(6):491-499, 1996.

Milder B, Rubin ML: *The fine art of prescribing glasses without making a spectacle of yourself,* Gainesville, Fla, Triad Scientific Publishers, 1991.

Magnification

The relative size of an image compared with its object is termed *magnification,* although the image may be larger or smaller than the object. Ophthalmologists must be aware of linear, axial, and angular magnification (Box 17-1).

TRANSVERSE MAGNIFICATION

Transverse magnification (also known as linear or lateral magnification) is used when the distances of the object and the image from the lens are known. Transverse magnification directly compares the *actual size* of the image to the *actual size* of the object. It does not deal with how big the image *looks* to an eye, but rather how big (or small) it is compared with the object. It refers to

Box 17-1 Types of Magnification

Transverse (lateral, linear)
Angular
Axial

the relative size of the image perpendicular to the optical axis of the lens system. Transverse magnification is thus defined as

Transverse magnification = image height/object height.

By similar triangles, the image height is related to the object height in the same proportion as the image distance to the object distance from the lens (Fig. 17-1). Thus the transverse magnification is

Transverse magnification = image height/object height

Image height/object height = image distance/object distance.

As illustrated in Fig. 17-2, if an object is located 50 cm to the left of a 5 D lens, the image will be located 33 cm (using the vergence formula, $-2 + 5 = 3$ D; $1/3$ D $= f = 0.3$ m or 33 cm) to the right of the lens. The transverse magnification can be calculated as

Image distance/object distance = 33 cm/50 cm = 0.67×

The image is thus two-thirds the size of the original object and is 33% smaller than the original.

There is often confusion about the nomenclature of magnification. An image that is magnified 3× is three times the size of the original object and is 200% larger. An image that is magnified 0.25× is one-quarter the size of the original object and is 75% smaller.

Clinical Example: Indirect Ophthalmoscopy

Transverse magnification can be used to calculate the magnification of the aerial image formed by the condensing lens in indirect ophthalmoscopy, as illustrated in

Fig. 17-3. For an emmetropic eye, the transverse magnification of the aerial image can be calculated as

Focal length of the lens/nodal point to retina distance = focal length of the lens/focal length of the eye in air = power of eye/power of lens.

Thus the transverse magnification of the image of the emmetropic eye (60 D) using a 20 D condensing lens is 60 ÷ 20 = 3×.

ANGULAR MAGNIFICATION

Angular magnification quantifies how large an image *appears* to the human eye. The object itself remains the same size, but as it is moved closer to the eye it subtends a larger visual angle and appears larger, and if it is moved away from the eye it subtends a smaller angle and appears smaller.

Angular magnification is a *comparison* of the visual angle that the image subtends at one distance compared with another. For example, consider an image that subtends 2° on a retina when the object is located 10 m from the eye. If the object is moved to 5 m from the eye, the

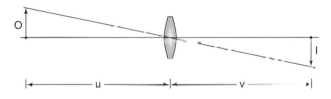

Fig. 17-1   The central ray and the optical axis form similar triangles. The ratio of the image height to the object height is the transverse magnification.

angular subtense will double and the image will appear twice as large as it did relative to when it was 10 m from the eye. Angular magnification *ALWAYS* requires that a reference distance be specified or assumed. Angular magnification is used with images and objects at infinity and when viewing objects with an eye.

Simple Magnifiers

With simple magnifiers, angular magnification compares the angular subtense produced by introduction of a lens to the angular subtense at a reference distance as shown in Fig. 17-4. By convention, that distance is 25 cm. Thus the angular magnification is

$$\text{Angular magnification} = \theta_{lens}/\theta_{25\ cm}.$$

For small angles, this can be simplified to

$$\text{Angular magnification} = \theta_{lens}/\theta_{25\ cm} \approx$$
$$\tan^{-1}(O/f) \div \tan^{-1}(O/25) \approx 25\ cm/4 = D/4.$$

The magnification of a lens used as a simple magnifier is the dioptric power of the lens divided by four.

Direct Ophthalmoscopy of the Emmetrope

During direct ophthalmoscopy, the examiner uses the power (60 D) of the emmetrope's eye as a simple magnifier, as illustrated in Fig. 17-5. Thus the emmetrope's fundus features appear 60 ÷ 4 = 15× larger than if the fundus had been cut out of the eye and held at a distance of 25 cm from the examiner's eye. The examination of an ametrope's fundus with a direct ophthalmoscope is a little bit more complicated and is discussed later under "Clinical Example: Direct Ophthalmoscopy of the Ametropic Fundus."

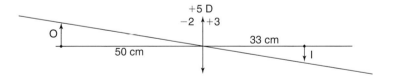

Fig. 17-2   An object is located 50 cm to the left of a +5 D lens and the image is formed 33 cm to the right of the lens.

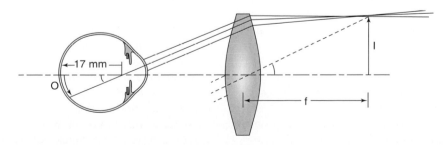

Fig. 17-3   An aerial image is formed by the condensing lens during indirect ophthalmoscopy.

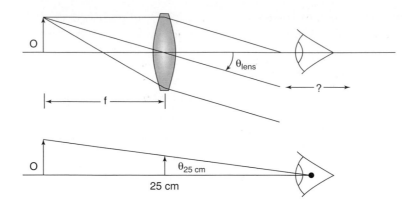

Fig. 17-4   The magnification produced by this plus lens used as a simple magnifier *(top)* is determined by comparing the angular size produced to the angular size produced at a reference distance (25 cm, *bottom*).

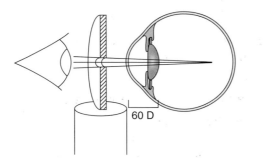

Fig. 17-5   An examiner uses the optics of the patient's eye as a simple magnifier to view the fundus.

Telescopes

Telescopes are optical devices consisting of two lenses (and objective and an eyepiece) that are precisely separated by the difference (Galilean) or sum (astronomical) of their focal lengths. When an object is viewed through a magnifying device such as a telescope, the angular magnification is the ratio of the angular subtense of the exiting rays compared with the angular subtense of the entering rays. Telescopes are usually used as magnifying devices, so the magnification is usually greater than 1×. Sometimes telescopes are used in "reverse," such that the angular subtense of the exiting rays is smaller and the magnification is less than 1× (for example 0.25×). For all telescopes, zero vergence in yields zero vergence out.

Astronomical telescopes   The astronomical, or Keplerian, telescope (Fig. 17-6) is composed of a plus power objective and a higher plus power eyepiece. The secondary focal point of the objective lens coincides with the primary focal point of the eyepiece; this is the intermediate image plane. Furthermore, the focal points co-incide in the intermediate image plane. The magnification is equal to

$$\text{Magnification} = \theta_{\text{out}} / \theta_{\text{in}} \approx f_{\text{objective}} / f_{\text{eyepiece}} = D_{\text{eyepiece}} / D_{\text{objective}}$$

An astronomical telescope forms an inverted image and thus has few uses in ophthalmic optics without the introduction of rectifying optical devices.

Galilean telescopes   A Galilean telescope (Fig. 17-7) is composed of a plus power objective and a higher power minus eyepiece. As in the astronomical telescope, the secondary focal point of the objective lens coincides with the primary focal point of the eyepiece lens. The focal points coincide in the intermediate image plane. The magnification is equal to

$$\text{Magnification} = \theta_{\text{out}} / \theta_{\text{in}} \approx f_{\text{objective}} / f_{\text{eyepiece}} = D_{\text{eyepiece}} / D_{\text{objective}}$$

just as in the astronomical telescope. In contrast, however, the Galilean telescope forms an upright image and is often used in ophthalmic optics. Furthermore, it should be noted that a 5× Galilean telescope composed of a −40 D eyepiece and a +8 D objective is shorter than a 5× astronomical telescope comprising a +40 D eyepiece and a +8 D objective (10 cm [Galilean] versus 15 cm [astronomical]).

Clinical example: surgical loupes   Surgical loupes are used for magnification in oculoplastic and strabismus surgery. They are almost always made of a Galilean telescope with an add to bring the far point to the surgeon's desired working distance.

Clinical example: direct ophthalmoscopy of the ametropic fundus   When the fundus of an ametropic eye is examined with a direct ophthalmoscope, lenses must be introduced to allow an emmetropic examiner to view the fundus. The lenses dialed into the head of the direct ophthalmoscope, in combination with the "error

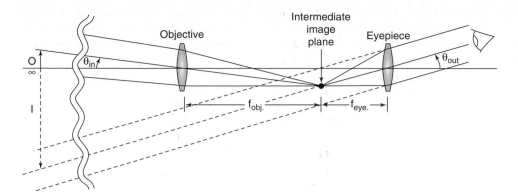

Fig. 17-6   An astronomical telescope.

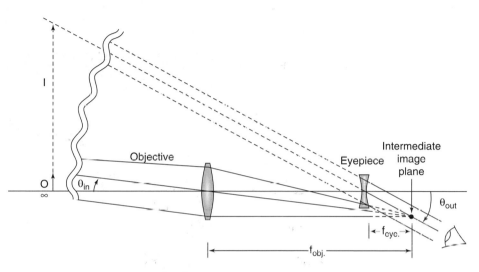

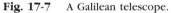

Fig. 17-7   A Galilean telescope.

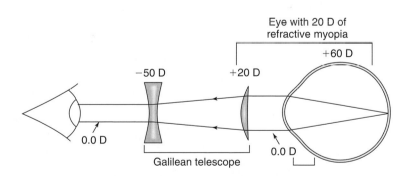

Fig. 17-8   An eye with 20 D of refractive myopia is viewed by an emmetropic examiner.

lens" of the ametropic patient's eye, form a Galilean telescope. This is illustrated in Fig. 17-8, in which the fundus of an eye with 20.00 D of refractive myopia (measured at the cornea) is viewed by an emmetropic observer. If the ophthalmoscope is 3 cm from the cornea, −50 D of power will be dialed into the ophthalmoscope. The patient's refractive error of +20 D (objective), combined with the −50 D (eyepiece), forms a Galilean telescope with a magnification of 50/20 = 2.5×. The fundus of this eye will appear 2.5× larger than if the eye were emmetropic. The *overall* magnification of the system, however, is the product of the magnification of the optics of the eye (60/4 = 15×) and the magnification of the telescope: 2.5 × 15 = 37.5×. Thus the fundus of this eye appears 37.5 times larger than if it were cut out of the eye and held 25 cm from the observer.

The minus power dialed into the direct ophthalmoscope, in combination with the plus power error lens of the myopic eye, forms a Galilean telescope that magnifies the view of the highly myopic fundus. The opposite is true for a hyperopic eye. The dioptric power of the hyperopic eye's optics is less than normal (a minus error lens), and plus power must be dialed into the ophthalmoscope to see the fundus clearly. This combination of lenses forms a "reverse" Galilean telescope and minifies the view of the fundus of the hyperopic eye. Other factors may also play a role in the apparent size of an optic nerve or retinal lesion, such as variations in true size (there is normal variation in the size of the optic nerve) or the presence of axial ametropia.

Summary

Telescopes and binoculars seem to bring known or familiar objects "closer" to us, because our mind has an idea of the object's size. Our brains tend to perceive a larger angular subtense for distant objects as "closer," although there are other clues (e.g., shadow or color overlap) that can modify that perception.

AXIAL MAGNIFICATION

Whereas transverse magnification refers to relative size *perpendicular* from the optical axis, axial magnification refers to the relative image size *along* the optical axis and is the square of the transverse magnification (Fig. 17-9):

Axial magnification = (transverse magnification)^2

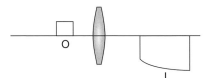
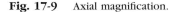

Fig. 17-9   Axial magnification.

The mathematical derivation of this formula is beyond the scope of this text, but its practical application is *mainly for indirect ophthalmoscopy*.

Clinical Example: Indirect Ophthalmoscopy

The condensing lens of the indirect ophthalmoscope produces an aerial image of the fundus above the condensing lens that can be observed by the examiner. Recall that the condensing lens produces a magnified image; the transverse magnification (for an emmetropic eye) of the aerial image is equal to the power of the eye (60 D) divided by the power of the condensing lens. As presented in the previous section, the axial magnification is the square of the transverse magnification.

Box 17-2   Magnification: Summary

TRANSVERSE MAGNIFICATION = IMAGE HEIGHT/OBJECT HEIGHT

Compares actual image size to actual object size
Does *not* convey how big an image looks to and eye
Use with objects and images at finite distances

ANGULAR MAGNIFICATION = $\theta_{out}/\theta_{in} \approx$ $f_{objective}/f_{eyepiece} = D_{eyepiece}/D_{objective}$ (TELESCOPES)

ANGULAR MAGNIFICATION = D/4 (SIMPLE MAGNIFIER)

Shows how large an image appears to an eye
Compares angular subtense of an object at two
    distances
Requires that a reference distance be specified or
    assumed
Use with objects and images at infinity (telescopes)
    and when viewing with an eye (simple magnifiers)

AXIAL MAGNIFICATION = (TRANSVERSE MAGNIFICATION)^2

Compares relative image size (depth) along the
    optical axis
Use with indirect ophthalmoscopy to determine image
    height/depth

Table 17-1   Comparison of magnification and depth distortion of the aerial image in indirect ophthalmoscopy of an emmetropic eye

Condensing lens power (D)	Transverse magnification	Axial magnification	Apparent axial magnification	Depth distortion
30	2×	4×	1×	0.50
20	3×	9×	2.25×	0.75
15	4×	16×	4×	1.00

However, eyepieces reduce the depth fourfold, so the apparent axial magnification is smaller, as detailed in Table 17-1.

Because of the "mismatch" between the apparent axial magnification and transverse magnification, higher power condensing lenses will reduce the apparent depth (or height) of a fundus anomaly compared with a + 15 D condensing lens.

Closing remarks The field of view in indirect ophthalmoscopy is *not* related to the power of the condensing lens, but rather to the diameter of the lens itself. The diameter of the condensing lens for a given lens power is limited by optical aberrations and other considerations that limit image quality. A larger diameter lens of the same power will have a larger field of view. The field of view for direct ophthalmoscopy is about 7°, whereas that for indirect ophthalmoscopy is about 25°. The exact

field of view, however, typically depends upon the size of the pupil (direct ophthalmoscopy) or the diameter of the condensing lens (indirect ophthalmoscopy).

SUMMARY

The important points to remember about the different types of and applications for magnification are presented in Box 17-2.

SUGGESTED READINGS

Rubin ML: *Optics for clinicians,* Gainesville, Fla, 1994, Triad Scientific Publishers.
Rubin ML, Walls GL: *Fundamentals of visual science,* Springfield, Ill, 1969, Charles C Thomas.

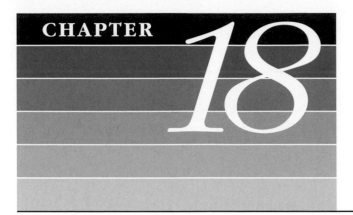

Aberrations of Spherical Lenses

No optical system behaves ideally, and the *aberrations* it produces affect image quality by deforming the image or by degrading its sharpness. Aberrations produced by the optics of the eye or by optical appliances (glasses, telescopes, or microscopes) can influence patient satisfaction with these appliances and with surgical procedures. The most clinically important aberrations in ophthalmology are chromatic aberration, spherical aberration, and astigmatism of oblique incidence.

CHROMATIC ABERRATION

Chromatic aberration results when multichromatic light is refracted by a lens. Recall that, for a given lens material, the index of refraction for blue wavelengths is higher than that for red. Thus shorter (blue) wavelengths are refracted more strongly than longer (red) ones (Fig. 18-1). This produces an axial chromatic interval of differently colored images along the optical axis of an optical system. Axial chromatic aberration is used to the advantage of the person performing refraction with the duochrome (bichrome) test. In addition, chromatic aberration produces colored fringes when a patient is viewing through the periphery of spectacle lenses and can be annoying, as discussed later in this chapter.

Clinical Applications

Duochrome (bichrome) test Because the human eye does not correct for chromatic aberration, the shorter wavelengths are focused closer to the lens than are the longer red ones (Fig. 18-2). In the emmetrope's eye, the retina is located about midway, dioptrically, between red and blue focal planes, corresponding to the focal area for yellow light. Although the full chromatic interval of the healthy human eye is about 1.25 to 1.5 D, the red and green filters commonly used in this test reduce it to about 0.5 D. The sphere endpoint of an ametrope's subjective refraction can be verified with the duochrome test.

Each eye is tested separately. A chart with targets on a red and green background is presented to a patient whose vision has been fogged by 0.5 to 0.75 D. The mild fogging helps to relax accommodation. If the patient was not overminused during the subjective refraction, he or she should be relatively myopic for a distance target. The patient should relate that the targets on the red background are clearer, and minus sphere should be added in 0.25 D increments until the targets on both sides are equally clear. If a patient reports that the targets on the green side are clearer, then plus sphere should be added until both sides are equally clear. Hence, the mnemonic, RAM-GAP: Red Add Minus—Green Add Plus. The test is then repeated for the fellow eye.

It is important to remember that the patient's visual acuity must be equal to or better than 20/30, because the 0.5 D difference between the red and green portions of the chart would not be discernible at a lesser acuity. In addition, this is a test involving chromatic aberration, not chromatic discrimination. Thus it can be successfully used in patients with congenital "color blindness." The duochrome test is summarized in Box 18-1.

Chromatic aberration of refractive and prism correction Spectacle lenses also produce chromatic aberration, which is particularly noticeable with higher power lenses. Lens materials with refractive indices that are similar for red and blue wavelengths are relatively free of chromatic aberration. A material with a larger

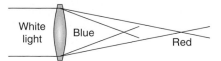

Fig. 18-1 Chromatic aberration. Shorter wavelength blue rays are refracted more strongly than longer wavelength red rays.

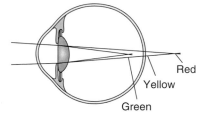

Fig. 18-2 Chromatic aberration of the eye.

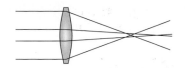

Fig. 18-3 Positive spherical aberration. Peripheral rays are more strongly refracted.

Box 18-1   Duochrome Test
Uses chromatic aberration of human eye to verify the spherical end point of the patient's subjective refraction
Is performed monocularly
Requires visual acuity of 20/30 or better
Can be used in patients with congenital "color blindness"

Table 18-1   Abbé values for common lens materials

Lens material	Refractive index	Abbé value
Crown glass	1.523	58
CR-39	1.498	48
SOLA Spectralite	1.537	47
Polycarbonate	1.586	30

difference in the indices of refraction for short and long wavelengths has more chromatic aberration. Although the derivation of the mathematical formulas describing it is beyond the scope of this text, the Abbé value of a lens material is a measure of its chromatic aberration (Table 18-1). The higher the Abbé value, the less chromatic aberration a lens produces. A lens material with a lower Abbé value is more likely to produce chromatic fringes, especially with higher power lenses. Note that lens materials with a lower index of refraction do not necessarily have higher Abbé values. Polycarbonate has a

higher index of refraction than that of CR-39, and although it is more impact resistant, it has a very low Abbé value.

Patients who require prism correction may also notice chromatic fringes around objects because of lateral chromatic aberration, but usually learn to accept the chromatic aberration in exchange for the relief from diplopia that the prism provides. The fringes are more noticeable with higher power prisms and with Fresnel Press-on prisms.

SPHERICAL ABERRATION

Rays that strike the paraxial portions of the lens are not focused to a point, and in positive spherical aberration they are focused closer to the lens, as shown in Fig. 18-3. The further away from the optical axis that a ray strikes the lens, the greater the spherical aberration.

Clinical Applications

Night myopia Spherical aberration accounts for much (but not all) of the phenomenon known as "night myopia." At low light levels, the pupil enlarges and allows more peripheral rays to enter the eye. The peripheral rays are focused anterior to the retina, rendering the eye relatively myopic in lower light levels. The typical amount of night myopia is about 0.5 D, but it can be as large as 1.25 D. Patients who are especially bothered by this phenomenon can be given two pairs of glasses (the second pair with more minus sphere for nighttime driving) or a clip-on spectacle with the necessary amount of sphere.

Retinoscopy in children Spherical aberration is also the basis for the "bulls eye" reflex seen in children during cycloplegic retinoscopy. When coming close to neutralization, the retinoscopist will observe "with" movement in the central portion of the pupil and "against" movement in the peripheral portions as the intercept is swept across the pupil. The reflex formed by the peripheral portions of the lens is relatively myopic and gives against movement while the central portion of the pupil is not yet neutralized. The central reflex should be the retinoscopist's endpoint to avoid underplussing. Overminusing (or underplussing) for an adult patient may lead to asthenopia, and in children it may lead to progression of myopia or an esodeviation.

ASTIGMATISM OF OBLIQUE INCIDENCE

Tilting a spherical lens adds sphere and cylinder of the same sign as the original lens and is called astigmatism of oblique incidence (Fig. 18-4). This phenomenon is also known as *radial astigmatism*. The effects of astigmatism of oblique incidence are more substantial with higher power lenses and greater amounts of tilt. About three times as much cylinder is induced relative to the amount of sphere, with its axis in the same meridian about which the lens is rotated. For example, tilting a +10.00 D lens 20° forward results in a lens with an effective power of $+10.41 + 1.38 \times 180$.

Clinical Applications

Pantoscopic tilt   To avoid astigmatism of oblique incidence, a spectacle lenses cannot be in the proper position for both straight-ahead gaze and downgaze. Frames are manufactured and the fit is adjusted so that there is a compromise between the two positions; this is termed *pantoscopic tilt*. The typical difference between straight ahead and the reading position is 15°, so the usual amount of pantoscopic tilt is 7.5°, with the lower edge of the spectacle frame being closer to the face than the top edge.

Myopes and tilted glasses   Myopes will sometimes tilt their glasses forward to gain more minus power, indicating a need for a stronger prescription. Tilting the lens forward induces both more minus sphere and minus cylinder, effectively increasing the minus spherical equivalent of the prescription. A hyperope could do the same to increase plus power, but will usually slide the glasses away from the eye (down the nose) to increase effective plus power via lens effectivity changes.

Corrected curve lenses   Spectacle lenses are also manufactured to reduce the amount of radial astigmatism (astigmatism of oblique incidence) they produce. In this case the front and back curves of a lens are designed to reduce this aberration.

Tilted intraocular lenses   Intraocular lenses (IOLs) with unstable fixation can have problems with tilt as well as with decentration. Decentration causes symptoms of glare and polyplopia. A tilted lens can induce a small amount of unanticipated power change, although the symptoms from decentration are usually more bothersome to the patient. Tilted IOLs are typically seen after surgery using scleral fixation techniques. An IOL of typical plus power tilted about its vertical axis would gain slight plus spherical power as well as plus cylinder at axis 90° relative to the eye. This would be *compensated for* by a small amount of minus sphere and cylinder in the refractive correction. In plus cylinder notation, the axis of the correcting cylinder would be at 180°; in minus cylinder notation it would be at 90°.

Off-axis measurement errors   Astigmatism of oblique incidence can also be a problem when one is attempting to objectively measure the refractive error of an eye. This is especially important when retinoscopy is performed on a patient who does not maintain fixation, as is commonly seen in small children. If a child looks to the side of the retinoscopist, the examiner would detect *correcting* plus cylinder at axis 180°.

SUGGESTED READING

Guyton DL, Uozato H, Wisnicki HJ: Rapid determination of intraocular lens tilt and decentration through the undilated pupil, *Ophthalmology* 97:1259-1264, 1990.

Rubin ML: *Optics for clinicians*, Gainesville, Fla, 1974, Triad Scientific Publishers.

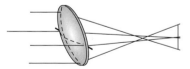

Fig. 18-4   Astigmatism of oblique incidence.

Contact Lenses

This chapter will discuss the optics and geometry of basic contact lens fitting, along with a few common-sense guidelines for evaluation of fit and complications. Contact lenses increase the field of vision relative to spectacle correction, especially for patients with aphakia, who are subject to ring scotomas when they wear spectacles. They also have an effect on image size; compared with spectacle lenses, minus power contact lenses produce less minification and plus power contact lenses produce less magnification. Thus, contact lenses can provide relief when there is symptomatic aniseikonia.

Spherical rigid contact lenses can be used to compensate for a toric anterior corneal surface. The "tear lens" effectively neutralizes the astigmatism induced by the toric anterior surface of the cornea. Irregular corneal surfaces (such as those seen after penetrating trauma or after radial keratotomy) that cause high and/or irregular astigmatism can be compensated for by a rigid contact lens, as long as a good fit can be obtained. In contrast, a soft contact lens generally conforms to the shape of the anterior corneal surface and will not neutralize corneal cylinder. If a soft contact lens is chosen for comfort, any significant astigmatism must be corrected by a toric lens. Despite the inability of soft contact lenses to correct corneal astigmatism, they are often preferred by patients because of comfort and by practitioners because of ease of fitting.

BASIC INFORMATION REQUIRED FOR CONTACT LENS FITTING

All patients who are to be fitted for contact lenses require a thorough slit lamp examination to detect conditions that might contraindicate wearing of contact lenses. In addition, keratometry readings and a good refraction are also necessary. The refractionist should measure vertex distance if significant ametropia is present (more than 5 D).

As previously discussed, the keratometer measures the radius of curvature of the anterior corneal surface by measuring the size of a reflected image. Although the keratometer *measures* the radius of curvature of the anterior corneal surface, the clinician is often more familiar with the dioptric power of the cornea, which is *calculated*. The dioptric scale on a keratometer assumes an "average" keratometric refractive index of 1.3375 that takes into account the minus power of the posterior surface of the cornea.

Contact lenses have a peripheral and a central radius of curvature. Keratometry (K) readings help the clinician to select the *base curve* of the contact lens. Because the power of the anterior corneal periphery is less than ("flatter," with a larger radius of curvature) that of the central cornea, different peripheral and central curves are needed for a well-fitting lens. The labeled base curve refers to the central posterior curve of the contact lens.

FITTING PARAMETERS

The basic fitting parameters of any contact lens are power, base curve, and diameter as detailed in Box 19-1. The power of a contact lens is determined by the refraction and vertex distance. The base curve and the diameter of a lens determine how well a lens will fit. A lens

---

Box 19-1   Contact Lens Parameters

Power, measured in diopters (D)
Base curve, measured in millimeters (mm)
Diameter, measured in millimeters (mm)

Box 19-2   Solutions for Contact Lens Fitting

IF A LENS IS TOO TIGHT:	IF A LENS IS TOO LOOSE:
Decrease diameter	Increase diameter
Flatten base curve	Steepen base curve

Box 19-3   Calculation of Rigid Contact Lens Power

1. Obtain K readings and refraction
2. Convert refraction to minus cylinder notation
   Disregard the minus cylinder, because it is corrected by the cylindrical tear lens
3. Convert the sphere power of the refraction to zero vertex distance
4. Choose a base curve for the contact lens that is slightly steeper (usually 0.5 D) than the flat K reading
   This forms a plus power spherical tear lens
5. Subtract the power of the spherical tear lens from the sphere value of the refraction to obtain the power of the contact lens

---

that fits well has sufficient movement to allow the flow of tears under the lens. If a lens has too little movement (too "tight"), the clinician should consider decreasing the diameter of the lens or flattening the base curve. If a lens is too "loose" (too much movement or the lens rides too high or too low), the diameter should be increased or the base curve should be steepened, as outlined in Box 19-2.

Soft lenses are readily available for "off-the-shelf" dispensing, but are generally available only in certain base curve and diameter combinations that are selected by the manufacturer. They are generally fit empirically, with the power determined by the overrefraction. Toric soft lenses are readily available, but fitting can be challenging, because some rotation of the lens (and the axis of the cylinder correction) occurs during each blink. Fit is evaluated by observing the movement of the lens during blink and by observing the patient in the office and during return visits.

Rigid lenses are also available in trial lens sets, with a variety of base curves and diameters. The choice of base curve is guided by the K readings and is usually selected to be slightly steeper than the flatter K reading to give a small apical clearance. Fit is evaluated by observation of the blink-induced excursion of the rigid lens and evaluation of the fluorescein pattern. The power of the rigid lens can be determined by refracting over a well-fitting rigid lens or by calculation as follows.

Clinical Application: Determination of Contact Lens Power

Consider a patient with the following refraction in the spectacle plane: $-11.25 + 1.25 \times 85$, with a vertex distance of 11 mm. The power of the contact lens can be determined by converting the prescription to minus cylinder notation:

$$-11.25 + 1.25 \times 85 \text{ becomes } -10.00 - 1.25 \times 175.$$

The minus power cylinder "tear lens" formed by the tears between the back of the contact lens and the front of the cornea will neutralize the corneal astigmatism and therefore can be dropped from the calculations. The -10.00 of sphere power is converted to zero vertex distance by combining the focal length of the correcting lens with the vertex distance:

$$10 \text{ cm} + 1.1 \text{ cm} = 11.1 \text{ cm}.$$

This is the focal length of the correcting lens at zero vertex distance. To obtain its power, take the reciprocal:

$$1/11.1 \text{ cm} = 1/0.111 \text{ m} = 9 \text{ D}.$$

Thus a rigid contact lens with a power of -9.00 D is required. However, many practitioners fit 0.5 D "steeper" than the flat K reading to give good apical clearance, so in this case a power of -9.50 D would be selected. The spherical tear lens of $+0.50$ D provides slight plus power. In this eye, the corneal cylinder is corrected by the minus cylindrical tear lens. The method for empirically determining contact lens power is summarized in Box 19-3.

RESIDUAL ASTIGMATISM

It should be noted that the astigmatism measured on retinoscopy or during subjective refraction is not always due to corneal shape considerations. The physician must be aware that lenticular astigmatism may exist in addition to or in isolation from corneal cylinder. Remember that the retina cannot cause astigmatism! The astigmatism that is measured with a spherical contact lens in place (assuming that it is not warped) is termed *residual astigmatism.* Residual astigmatism can be predicted by comparing the refraction in the spectacle plane with the K readings.

Clinical Application: Anticipating Residual Astigmatism

Consider an eye with K readings of 42.00/43.50@90. If one assumes that there is no lenticular astigmatism, this amount of corneal astigmatism would be corrected by a +1.50 cylinder × 90 or a −1.50 cylinder × 180, in addition to any spherical correction. If the spectacle correction was −2.00 + 1.50 × 90 (−0.50 − 1.50 × 180), no residual astigmatism would be anticipated when a rigid spherical contact lens was worn.

With the same K readings and a spectacle refraction of −3.00 + 0.50 × 90, residual astigmatism should be anticipated. In this eye with K readings of 42.00/43.50@90 and a spectacle refraction of −3.00 + 0.50 × 90, 1 D of the corneal astigmatism is negated by the presence of 1 D of lenticular astigmatism. In this case, a spherical soft contact lenses would be a good choice, because a rigid lens would unmask the lenticular astigmatism.

CONTACT LENSES AND MAGNIFICATION

Compared with spectacles, minus power contact lenses produce less minification and plus power contact lenses produce less magnification than spectacle correction. The difference in magnification in spectacle or contact lenses can be used optically to help symptoms in selected situations. For instance, a person with high hyperopia and mild-to-moderate visual impairment who has contact lens correction may be happier with the image magnification afforded by a change to spectacle correction. Contact lenses can provide relief when there is symptomatic aniseikonia, as discussed in the following example.

Clinical Application

A person with monocular aphakia corrected with a +12.00 D spectacle lens will have about 24% magnification relative to the other eye, which will prevent fusion. The spectacle-corrected aphakic eye can be modeled, using the error lens concept, as a reverse Galilean telescope with added minus power in the eye (the eyepiece)

and the correcting plus spectacle lens (the objective) in front of the eye. The magnification produced by aphakic eye/aphakic spectacle correction can be decreased by fitting an aphakic contact lens. However, even an aphakic contact lens produces some magnification, which may be bothersome to the patient. Aniseikonia produced by monocular aphakia can be helped by constructing a *reverse* Galilean telescope as follows (remember that if one looks "backward" through a telescope things look smaller). The power of the aphakic contact lens can be increased ("overplussed") to leave the patient myopic at distance. The aphakic contact lens-induced myopia is then "treated" with a minus spectacle lens. The overplussed contact lens and the minus power spectacle lens form a reverse Galilean telescope. (An added point is that preexisting axial myopia [or a scleral buckle] would further increase the residual magnification of contact lens-corrected aphakia.)

CONTACT LENSES AND ACCOMMODATION

Myopic eyes must accommodate *more* with contact lens correction than with spectacle lens correction. From an optical standpoint, contact lens correction eliminates the accommodative advantage of spectacles for myopia and the disadvantage of spectacles for hyperopia.

Clinical Application

One should use caution when fitting contact lenses for a myope with spectacle correction who is likely to be nearing development of presbyopia. This person will leave the office with excellent distance vision, and later will discover that his or her near vision is poorer with contact lenses than with glasses. The individual may believe that your contact lens fitting or the drops you used during the examination caused difficulty with near vision.

SUGGESTED READINGS

Basic and clinical science course: section 3, San Francisco, 2001, American Academy of Ophthalmology.

Contact lenses: the CLAO guide to basic science and clinical practice, ed 3, Metairie, LA, 1995, The Contact Lens Association of Ophthalmologists.

The CLAO pocket guide to contact lens fitting, Metairie, La, The Contact Lens Association of Ophthalmologists.

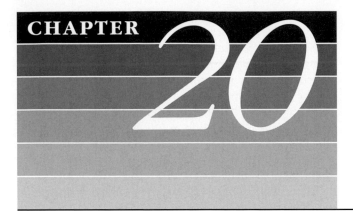

Assessment of Vision

Although ophthalmologists usually think of "reading the letters" when visual acuity is measured, letter recognition acuity is not the only type of measurement that quantifies human visual function. Snellen acuity is one type of minimum resolvable acuity. Other types of visual acuity are minimum visible and spatial minimum discriminable. Some other parameters also contribute to visual function, including the amount of light, the contrast, the refractive state of the eye, and the health of the visual system.

TYPES OF VISUAL ACUITY

The three major types of visual acuity are minimum visible, minimum resolvable, and minimum discriminable, as summarized in Table 20-1. Each evaluates a different aspect of visual function and has a different threshold.

Minimum visible acuity is the determination of the presence or absence of a visual stimulus, for example, the presence or absence of a line on a uniform visual field. This type of acuity depends not on the size of the cone cell (20 seconds of arc), but on differences in local brightness. In this type of acuity determination, the subject is not asked to make any spatial differentiation, but only to judge the presence or absence of a visual stimulus.

Minimum resolvable acuity (also known as minimum separable, minimum legible, or ordinary visual acuity) is the type of acuity most familiar to ophthalmologists. Ordinary Snellen acuity is measured with high-contrast letters or figures understandable to the subject. Unfortunately, not all letters of the alphabet are equally difficult to recognize, so charts have been developed that use font selection and letter selection to minimize this problem. An example of this is the ETDRS chart. The ETDRS chart is also known as the Ferris-Bailey distance visual acuity chart and uses only 10 letters. Other optotype tests, including the tumbling E and the Landolt C, are also available. The Landolt C test is the international standard and is administered such that the subject is asked to tell whether the gap in the C is facing up, right, left, or down. Grating acuity is also an example of minimum resolvable acuity, but it is unfamiliar to many subjects and is prone to guessing errors if there is a binary choice for identification of the orientation of the gratings.

Spatial minimum discriminable, also known as vernier acuity or hyperacuity, is the ability of the eye to detect subtle offset or misalignment of two lines. The human eye is capable of discerning offsets (3 to 5 seconds of arc) that are smaller to the diameter of the human cone (20 seconds of arc). The physiologic mechanism for this is still not understood.

MEASURING AND RECORDING VISUAL ACUITY

Visual acuity should be tested monocularly with the proper refractive correction in place and should be measured at distance and near. In certain circumstances it may also be necessary to record the uncorrected acuity. In patients with an assumed head posture (from nystagmus), it is also important to measure the acuity in their posture and in the forced primary position.

Table 20-1   Types of visual acuity and threshold

Acuity	Threshold
Minimum visible	1-10 seconds of arc
Minimum resolvable (minimum separable, minimum legible, or ordinary visual acuity)	30-60 seconds of arc
Minimum discriminable (spatial minimum discriminable, hyperacuity, or vernier acuity)	3-5 seconds of arc

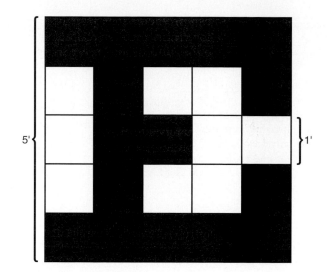

Fig. 20-1   A Snellen "E." Each element of the E subtends 1 minute of visual angle.

Table 20-2   Visual acuity notation

Snellen acuity		Snellen fraction	MAR
Feet	Meters		
20/10	6/3	2.0	0.5
20/20	6/6	1.0	1.0
20/25	6/7.5	0.8	1.25
20/30	6/9	0.67	1.5
20/40	6/12	0.5	2.0
20/50	6/15	0.4	2.5
20/60	6/18	0.33	3.0
20/80	6/24	0.25	4.0
20/100	6/30	0.2	5.0
20/120	6/36	0.17	6.0
20/150	6/45	0.133	7.5
20/200	6/60	0.10	10.0
20/400	6/120	0.05	20.0

The eye not to be tested is usually occluded while the fellow eye is tested. However, in individuals with manifest and/or latent nystagmus it is essential to test acuity while "fogging" the untested eye. Usually this means using a +6.00 to +8.00 D lens over the eye that is not being tested. Occluding the untested eye of a person with nystagmus often leads to an increase in the amplitude of the nystagmus and a commensurate decrease in visual acuity. In persons with nystagmus, binocular acuity should also be recorded, because it is often significantly better that monocular acuity and is more representative of physiologic conditions. This can be especially important to an individual with nystagmus who may be eligible for a driver's license.

The Snellen fraction is the most common notation used to record minimum resolvable acuity. Each element of a Snellen E subtends 1 minute of visual angle, and the entire Snellen E subtends 5 minutes in height and width (Fig. 20-1) at a specified test distance. Thus a Snellen fraction of 20/60 means that at 20 feet a letter can be seen that subtends 5 minutes of arc when viewed at 60 feet. The numerator denotes the test distance, and the denominator notes the test distance at which the letter would subtend a visual angle of 5 minutes. Acuity recorded in metric fashion usually uses a numerator of 6 m.

By definition, a 20/20 size E subtends a visual angle of 5 minutes when viewed at 20 feet. In concrete terms, this E measures about 9 mm in height and width, with each leg and space measuring about 1.75 mm. Accordingly, a 20/200 size E measures about 9 cm in height and width. A 20/200 size E is *roughly* equivalent to the size of *some* examiners' hands.

The minimum angle of resolution (MAR) is an alternative method to record acuity and is used in many large clinical studies in which visual acuity is an outcome measure. In MAR notation, 20/20 acuity would equal 1 minute, 20/40 acuity would equal 2 minutes, etc., as shown in Table 20-2. When statistical analysis is necessary to compare acuity outcome, the logarithm of the MAR (logMAR) is used. Charts for logMAR have an equal number of letters in each row, with a geometric progression of decreasing sizes of letters and spaces. These charts are too large to be readily projected for larger size optotypes, so the patient with lesser acuity must be moved closer to the chart for testing and the acuity recalculated accordingly.

Near acuity is also measured when the patient has the best refractive correction in place and a reading addition if necessary. Both the size of the optotype read and the testing distance must be recorded: "OD J8 at 6 inches; OS J1+ at 14 inches."

FACTORS AFFECTING VISUAL ACUITY

Numerous factors can affect visual acuity, and a partial list is given in Box 20-1. Uncorrected refractive errors

---

Box 20-1 Factors Adversely Affecting Visual Acuity

Young or old age
Large (>6) or small (<2.5 mm) pupil size
Decreased contrast
Uncorrected refractive error
Eccentric viewing
Ocular and visual pathway disease

Box 20-2 Testing Visual Acuity in Children

Blinks to light
Fix and follow
Central, steady, and maintained
Pictures
Lea symbols
HOTV
Illiterate E's
Landolt C's
Numbers
Snellen letters

---

lead to optical degradation of the image on the retina. Eccentric viewing (as with amblyopia or a macular scar) also leads to poor visual acuity because of the absence of proper retinal anatomy for high-resolution acuity. When contrast is reduced, there is a reduction of acuity, even in the healthy eye. Small or large pupils also limit acuity because of diffraction. Finally, ocular and visual pathway disease may also limit visual acuity.

DEVELOPMENT OF VISUAL ACUITY

Babies are born with an immature visual system and do not have the visual acuity, color discrimination, visual fields, or eye movement control of adults. Visual function develops rapidly, especially during the first 6 months of life. At birth, the visual response may be recorded as "blinks to light," although some infants with normal vision will seem more or less visually alert than their contemporaries. "Fix and follow" vision develops during the first 3 months of age, and an infant should have central, steady, and maintained vision by 6 months of age.

Although it is not possible, strictly speaking, to measure optotype acuity in an infant or preverbal child, forced preferential looking (FPL) and visual evoked potentials (VEPs) have been used to estimate visual acuity in infants and investigate the development of visual function. At birth, the acuity is around 20/400, and it improves to 20/100 as measured by FPL and 20/30 as measured by VEPs by 6 months of age.

TESTING VISUAL ACUITY IN CHILDREN

As noted in the preceding section, the clinical visual response is noted as blinks to light, fix and follow, or central steady and maintained in infancy. FPL or VEPs can also be used if available to the clinician and the clinical condition mandates that a formal or quantitative measure of visual acuity is necessary. Even when these tests are performed by a skilled examiner, their usefulness is partially affected by the cooperation and attention span of the child. Any difference in the objection to covering of either eye should be noted, as this may indicate amblyopia.

When a preverbal pediatric patient with amblyopia has strabismus, it is easy to tell which eye the patient prefers to fix with and therefore to judge whether significant amblyopia is present. The ability of the amblyopic eye to hold fixation when the sound eye is covered is indicative of the severity of the amblyopia. When a pediatric patient with straight eyes has amblyopia, the examiner can use the induced tropia test. In this test a base-down prism is placed before one eye, which induces a hypertropia. The power of the prism should be high enough to be able to see the fixation switch, but not so high that the acuity of the eye behind the prism is degraded; a 15 to 20Δ prism usually works well. The examiner places it before one eye and then the other and observes the fixation preference of the child.

When the child can speak or can cooperate with matching games, acuity can be measured with optotypes more familiar to the clinician. The most difficult test for which the child's cooperation can be reliably obtained should be used. Methods to test visual acuity in infants and children are shown in Box 20-2. Linear (more than one figure on a line) optotypes are always preferred because of the crowding phenomenon (see the next section). Measurement with isolated optotypes may overestimate the visual acuity and may make it difficult to diagnose amblyopia.

CROWDING PHENOMENA

The crowding phenomenon is important in the measurement of visual acuity in individuals with amblyopia. They have difficulty judging offset in tests of vernier acuity and difficulty separating closely spaced objects. Thus the crowding effect describes the fact that the individual with amblyopia will have better acuity with single letters

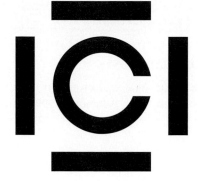

Fig. 20-2   "Crowded" optotype (Landolt C with crowding bars).

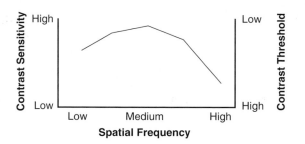

Fig. 20-3   Normal contrast sensitivity curve.

than with linear or "crowded" optotypes (Fig. 20-2). Individuals with strabismic amblyopia are especially prone to exhibiting the crowding effect. The crowding phenomenon also causes optotype acuity to be worse than grating acuity.

Amblyopic eyes exhibit decreased contrast sensitivity in addition to decreased optotype acuity, especially at higher spatial frequencies (see the next section on "Contrast Sensitivity"). The visual deficits in amblyopia affect primarily foveal function, and the amblyopic eye appears to have receptive fields that are inappropriately large in the foveal visual cortex.

CONTRAST SENSITIVITY

Snellen and typical optotype acuity is measured with high contrast (approaching 100%), but daily tasks are frequently carried out at much lower levels of contrast. Ocular and visual pathway diseases may drastically reduce visual function, while the physician measures normal or near-normal visual acuity. One way to quantify that loss is with contrast sensitivity testing. Contrast sensitivity testing is still evolving, and some controversy exists as to what is the optimal and most efficient way to measure contrast sensitivity.

Tests of contrast sensitivity are administered when the patient has the best refractive correction in place and with normal room illumination and with the pupils in their natural state. Two main types of contrast sensitivity tests are in common use today: those that use sine waves and those that use optotypes. Tests that use sine wave gratings (e.g., the Vistech chart) present different orientations of the gratings (vertical, tilt right, and tilt left) with progressively less contrast over a range of grating sizes. A plot is made of the minimum resolvable contrast target at a variety of spatial frequencies (Fig. 20-3). A contrast sensitivity function is plotted over a range of spatial frequencies. Tests that use optotypes (e.g., the Pelli-Robson test) generate a similar plot using optotypes

of diminishing size and contrast. This type of test has the advantage that it may be easier for some patients to comprehend and is more similar to real life situations.

In either case, certain ocular diseases tend to affect different portions of the contrast sensitivity function (CSF) preferentially. Optic nerve disease and glaucoma tend to decrease contrast sensitivity in the middle of the curve. Refractive errors, macular disease, corneal pathologic conditions, and amblyopia seem to affect the CSF at higher spatial frequencies. Cataracts affect both portions of the CSF.

Contrast sensitivity testing is an increasingly important method used to quantify visual function both in clinical practice and in research protocols.

PINHOLE ACUITY TESTING

A pinhole aperture increases the depth of focus of the eye and reduces the size of blur circles. During visual acuity testing, a pinhole can compensate for small amounts of refractive error and allow assessment of visual acuity without refractive correction in place. A 1.2 mm pinhole is most effective for "neutralizing" refractive errors (up to 3 D). Smaller pinholes increase diffraction and decrease the amount of light entering the eye; larger ones do not compensate for as much refractive error. For example, a 2 mm pinhole is easier for some patients to use, but it can only "neutralize" 1 D of refractive error. Thus, when larger refractive errors are known or suspected to be present (e.g., aphakia), the majority of the refractive correction should be placed in the trial frame behind the pinhole.

Clinical Application

Occluders with multiple pinhole apertures are easier for some patients to use. Patients with tremors may be unable to hold pinholes steady enough with their hand for the pinhole acuity test to be effective, but the test may be able to be used if the pinhole is mounted in a spectacle (in a trial lens frame or a lens clip over their glasses).

Pinhole acuity can also be used to help identify the cause of visual loss or complaints. If, with the best refractive correction in place, the patient complains of unsatisfactory vision, a pinhole placed over the refractive correction may aid in the diagnosis. If the acuity improves, this suggests a media problem (corneal or lenticular); if the acuity drops with the pinhole, this is more suggestive of a retinal etiology.

SUGGESTED READINGS

Guyton DL, West CE, Miller JM, Wisnicki HJ: *Ophthalmic optics and clinical refraction,* Baltimore, 1999, Prism Press.

Hart WM: *Adler's physiology of the eye,* St Louis, 1992, Mosby.

CHAPTER 21

Physical Optics

No one theory of light can explain its interaction with all materials. The description of light's interaction with matter is divided into geometric optics, physical optics, and quantum optics.

Geometric optics models light as rays and is used to understand the imaging properties of lens systems; it ignores the effects of diffraction and other physical phenomena, but is still useful to allow us to model optical systems. Although geometric optics helps us to understand the behavior of light rays, it does not describe the interaction between light and matter. Physical optics describes the properties of light's interaction with matter that are most easily understood using wave theory, whereas quantum optics treats light as having both wave and photon characteristics. This chapter will summarize and categorize the wave and particle characteristics of light and some applications in ophthalmology.

WHAT IS LIGHT?

Visible light is but a small portion of the electromagnetic spectrum (Fig. 21-1) and is defined as that part of the electromagnetic spectrum with a wavelength between 400 and 700 nm. Although light has both an electric and a magnetic field, the magnetic aspects are usually disregarded in physical optics.

The speed of light in a vacuum (c) is constant and is equal to 3.00×10^{10} cm/s. The frequency of light, υ, is related to the wavelength, λ, by the following equation:

$$c = \upsilon\lambda$$

Thus, as the wavelength (units = cm) shortens, the frequency (units s^{-1}) increases, and, conversely, as the wavelength increases, the frequency decreases.

When light leaves a vacuum and enters a transparent medium, it slows down—the velocity decreases. As discussed in Chapter 11, the ratio of the speed of light in a vacuum (c) to the speed of light in a medium (v) is the refractive index (n) of that medium:

$$n = c/v$$

Because light always travels faster in a vacuum than in a material, the refractive index of a material is always greater than 1. In addition, the refractive index of a material is slightly different for each wavelength of light. For example, the refractive index of air for violet light (436 nm) is 1.0002957, and for red light (656 nm) it is 1.0002914. Refractive indices for ophthalmic materials are usually given for yellow light unless stated otherwise. When light enters a new medium, the frequency of the light does not change, but the wavelength does. The simplest case is when light travels from a vacuum to a transparent medium; the wavelength shortens in the new medium.

PHOTON PROPERTIES OF LIGHT

When light interacts with a material, light may be emitted or absorbed if the conditions are correct. The amount of energy (E) in a photon is described by $E = h\upsilon$, where υ is frequency of the light wave and h is Planck's constant (6.62×10^{-34}). Because, by definition, blue light has a higher frequency than red light, photons from

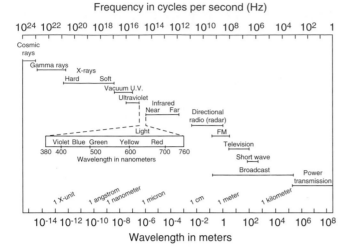

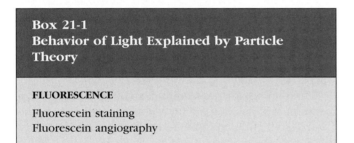

Fig. 21-1   The electromagnetic spectrum, with the visible portion expanded.

Table 21-1	Behavior of light explained by wave properties
Principle	**Ophthalmic application**
Interference	Antireflection films
	Interference films
	Laser interferometry to test retinal function
Polarization	Polarized sunglasses
	Crossed polarizers in ophthalmic instruments
	Haidinger brushes
	Sensory testing—stereopsis and suppression
Diffraction	Limits visual acuity with small pupil size
	Diffractive multifocal IOLs and contact lenses
Reflection	Specular microscopy
	Inversely proportional to λ^4
Scattering	Explains flare in anterior chamber
	Blue sky
	Red sunsets
	Corneal haze with corneal edema

Box 21-1
Behavior of Light Explained by Particle Theory

FLUORESCENCE
Fluorescein staining
Fluorescein angiography

---

blue light have more energy than those from longer wavelengths.

Clinical Application: Fluorescein

During fluorescein angiography, an excitation filter is used to produce 480 nm blue light. The blue light is absorbed by the fluorescein molecule, which in turn emits lower-energy yellow-green light between 500 and 600 nm with a peak at 520 nm. A "barrier" filter is used on the exiting light to capture emitted light of longer wavelengths more effectively. Thus, fluorescein angiography and fluorescein staining are best understood using the photon aspects of light, as summarized in Box 21-1.

WAVE PROPERTIES OF LIGHT

Two of the principal characteristics of a wave are its amplitude and its wavelength and the third is its frequency. Several commonly observed ophthalmic phenomena and applications are best described by understanding the wave properties of light, shown in Table 21-1.

Interference and Coherence

Because of the wave nature of light, distinct waves can interact with each other in a constructive fashion (when they are in phase) or a destructive fashion (when they are out of phase). Coherence is the ability of two light beams from the same source to produce interference. Spatial coherence is the ability of two separate portions of the same wave to produce interference, as shown in Fig. 21-2. Slits can be placed to produce spatially coherent light, resulting in a series of light and dark bands corresponding to areas of constructive and destructive interference, respectively.

Temporal coherence is the ability of one wave to interfere with another wave in the same light beam. Temporally coherent light can be produced by selecting a filter that permits only a narrow band of wavelength to be transmitted through the filter.

Clinical application: antireflection films/coatings Antireflection coatings, illustrated in Fig. 21-3, are frequently applied to spectacle and ophthalmic lenses to reduce unwanted reflections from the lens surface. Most antireflection coatings consist of several thin layers of transparent materials, designed to reduce reflections in the visible spectrum, and the index of refraction of the coating must be less than that of the lens material. A thin coating one-quarter wavelength thick is applied to the lens surface. If the coating has the proper index of refraction, equal quantities of light waves are reflected from both the air-coating interface and the coating-lens

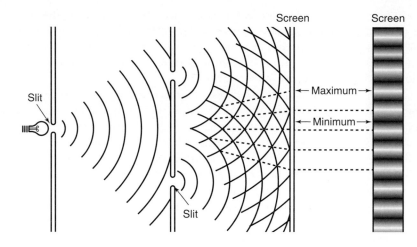

Fig. 21-2   Slits are used to create spatially coherent light. The light bands correspond to areas of constructive interference and the dark bands correspond to destructive interference.

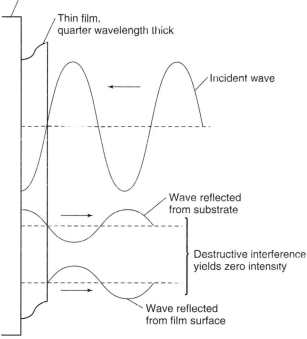

Fig. 21-3   Antireflection coating. The two reflected beams are equal in amplitude, but one-half wavelength out of phase with each other, producing destructive interference and reducing reflection from the lens surface.

interface. The waves reflected from the front and back surfaces of the coating are exactly one-half wavelength out of phase and thus destructively interfere with each other. With carefully manufactured coatings, the overall reflection from a lens surface can be reduced from 4% to 5% to less than 1%.

Clinical application: interference filters in fluorescein angiography   During fluorescein angiography, an "excitation filter" allows only light with a narrow band of wavelengths around 480 nm (blue light) to stimulate and

excite the fluorescein molecule and illuminate the eye. The radiation spectrum of the fluorescein molecule is between 500 and 600 nm, although the peak is close to 520 nm. A barrier filter that transmits only temporally light with a wavelength close to 520 nm blocks the other (excitation) wavelengths from striking the film.

Clinical application: interference fringes as a test of retinal function   Another important application of interference is laser interferometry, for which interference patterns are projected onto the retina to measure grating visual acuity. A laser beam is split into two beams that enter the eye through different portions of the pupil. Where the beams overlap on the retina, interference fringes are produced, and the grating visual acuity can be determined by changing the separation of the interfering beams. Interference fringes are not substantially degraded by a cataractous lens, so retinal function can be assessed before cataract surgery.

Polarization

Unpolarized light consists of waves with a random orientation of electrical planes, in contrast to polarized light, which consists of waves that all have their electrical planes in the same direction. Polarized light can be produced by passing a beam of unpolarized light through a polarizing filter and can be used to produce light that is linearly (plane), circularly, or elliptically polarized. Linearly (plane) polarized light is the easiest to envision. Imagine a taut rope that is snapped, generating a sinusoidal wave. Now imagine a collection of ropes with a variety of orientations of the waves—this is similar to unpolarized light. Using the same analogy, now imagine that the same collection of ropes were passed through vertical slits in a picket fence; only those waves that were oriented parallel to the slits in the picket fence would pass through the fence. These waves would be linearly polarized in the vertical direction.

Sunlight consists of a mixture of polarized and unpolarized light. Direct sunlight is unpolarized, but when it encounters a surface, the reflected sunlight will be partially polarized. The amount of polarization that occurs depends on the material and the incident angle of the light.

Clinical application: polarized sunglasses The amount of polarization that occurs during outdoor activities depends on the material and the incident angle of the light. When a person is boating, the sunlight reflected from the surface of the water is partially polarized, especially in the horizontal direction. A similar situation occurs when a person is driving toward the sun—the light reflected from the road surface is strongly polarized parallel to the road. Vertically polarized sunglasses can reduce the amount of light reflected from the water's or road's surface.

Clinical application: sensory testing Plane polarized lenses can be used to evaluated stereopsis and suppression. Plane polarized filters are placed before each eye at 90° to each other, and targets are presented that are also polarized and visible to only the left or right eye. Stereopsis tests often use polarized lenses. Similar tests are also available for testing at distance to evaluate the presence and depth of suppression in intermittent exotropia.

Clinical application: ophthalmic instruments Some ophthalmic instruments use polarizing lenses in an attempt to eliminate glare from the light reflected from the cornea. The examiner views the patient's eye through a polarized filter that is polarized opposite to the light used to illuminate the area of interest. Glare is reduced, but often at the expense of reduced illumination and unusual ophthalmoscopic and retinoscopic reflexes. Using a polarizing retinoscope to perform retinoscopy in a child with well-dilated eyes produces an unusual Maltese cross-like reflex that is difficult to see and to accurately determine "with" and "against" movement.

Clinical application: Haidinger brushes phenomenon The human eye is not ordinarily sensitive to the polarization of light, with the exception of the Haidinger brushes phenomenon. This phenomenon is demonstrated by viewing a blue light source through a rotating linearly (plane) polarized filter. A "propeller" or double-ended brush is seen rotating as the filter rotates. Historically, this test was used to assess macular function through dense cataracts before cataract surgery was recommended or to detect eccentric fixation in an amblyopic eye.

Diffraction

When a light wave encounters an aperture, obstruction, or irregularity, it changes direction and seems to "bend around" the edge of the aperture. Light and dark bands, called diffraction patterns, are seen in the geometric shadow of the edge of the aperture. Diffraction can only occur when light passes by an opaque edge, but it seldom occurs without other phenomena such as interference or refraction.

When the aperture is large relative to the size of the wavelength, diffraction does not substantially limit the resolution of the optical system. However, diffraction can become significant with smaller apertures and at the edges of larger ones. Shorter wavelengths are less subject to diffraction than are longer wavelengths. A small circular aperture, such as a small pupil, will produce a diffraction pattern with a small circular bright disk (the Airy disk), surrounded by halos of alternating dark and light. Diffraction can limit visual acuity when the pupil is less than 2.5 mm.

Clinical application: diffractive lenses Multifocal contact lenses and intraocular lenses (IOLs) can be manufactured as diffractive lenses, where a series of radial steps or zones of decreasing width are etched onto the surface of the lens, similar to the lines on a Fresnel prism. The light diffracted by the steps creates a second focal point for that portion of the lens. Although diffractive IOLs are gaining in popularity, the multifocal properties come at the expense of reduced contrast sensitivity, and they may not be suitable for individuals who require optimal contrast sensitivity, particularly in low-light situations.

Reflection

When light encounters an interface that divides two media with different indices of refraction, not all of the light is refracted, and some (or nearly all, in some cases) is reflected. The amount of light that is reflected is proportional in large part to the difference in refractive index and to a certain extent to the angle of incidence.

Clinical applications: keratometry The air-tear interface reflects about 2% of the light incident on the human eye and is responsible for the corneal light reflex, also known as the first Purkinje–Sanson image. Illuminated rings can also be reflected from the eye and are used to measure the radius of curvature of the anterior corneal surface (keratometry).

Clinical application: specular microscopy Specular microscopy can be used to examine the corneal endothelium. Contact or noncontact techniques are available, but both use separate illumination and viewing paths so that the reflection from the anterior corneal surface does not interfere with the reflection from the endothelial cell/aqueous interface. The light that is dimly reflected from the endothelial surface can be collected for quantification of endothelial cell density and morphology.

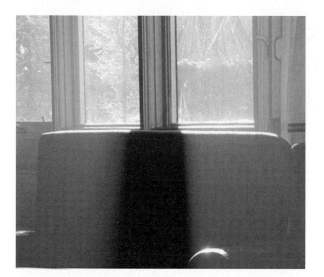

Fig. 21-4   Sunlight entering a smoky room; the light is scattered by particles in the air.

SCATTERING

Scattering is related to both diffraction and to reflection and occurs when light encounters irregularities in the light path, such as molecules or particles. Scattering is evident in a theater where dust is in the air and the projector beam is viewed from the side, as demonstrated in Fig. 21-4.

Clinical application: the blue sky and the red sunset When the particles are small relative to the wavelength of light, such as when light from the sun encounters the molecules in our atmosphere, *Rayleigh scattering* occurs. The intensity of the scattering is *inversely* proportional to λ^4, that is, wavelength to the fourth power. Thus, shorter wavelengths are scattered more than longer (red) ones. The light from the sky appears blue because of this phenomenon. The blue rays are scattered (more than the longer ones) by the gas molecules in the atmosphere, making the sky appear blue. Rayleigh scattering also accounts for the red sunset. As the sun approaches the horizon, more and more of the shorter rays are scattered (and lost), leaving only the longest (red) ones to stimulate the retina.

Clinical application: slit lamp beam The "optical section" formed by the slit lamp beam is a result of scattering by the ocular tissues, as is the flare caused by proteins in the aqueous humor. Scattering can interfere with vision and can cause glare when light encounters irregularities in the cornea or lens. Scattering also reduces contrast and degrades image detail on the retina.

TRANSMISSION AND ABSORPTION

Transmission is the amount of light energy that passes through a medium, and is quantified in terms of transmittance, the percentage of energy that passes through it. Lenses can be designed to absorb light energy to optimize visual function.

Clinical Application: Absorptive Lenses

Dark sunglasses absorb up to 90% of incident light in order to improve comfort and to improve dark adaptation after exposure to bright outdoor lighting. They can also reduce unwanted glare. Ultraviolet absorbency lenses can protect the eye from its potentially damaging effects. Ultraviolet light is thought to cause or contribute to the formation of actinic keratopathy and cortical cataracts.

SUGGESTED READING

Rubin ML, Walls GL: *Fundamentals of visual science,* Springfield, Ill, 1969, Charles C Thomas.

CHAPTER 22

Summary of Important Equations and Relationships

VERGENCE FORMULA

$$U + D = V.$$

where U = the vergence of the light entering the lens (D), D = the vergence contributed by the lens (the lens power) (D), and V = the vergence of the light leaving the lens (D).

FOCAL LENGTH OF A LENS

$$f = 1/D,$$

where f = focal length of the lens (m) and D = power of the lens (D).

POWER OF A SPHERICAL REFRACTING SURFACE

$$D_s = |n' - n|/r,$$

where D = power of the surface, in diopters, n = refractive index, and r = radius of curvature, in meters.

MAGNIFICATION

Spectacle Lens Magnification

$M_{spectacle\ lens}$ = 2% per diopter of spectacle lens power (assumes 12 mm vertex distance).

Transverse Magnification

$M_{transverse}$ = image height/object height = image distance/object distance.

• Compares actual image size to actual object size.
• Does *not* convey how big an image looks to and eye.
Transverse magnification is used with objects and images at finite distances.

Angular Magnification

• Shows how large an image appears to an eye.
• Compares the angular subtense of an object at two distances.
• Requires that a reference distance be specified or assumed.

Type	Vergence added by surface is	Image of real object is
Plano	None, just reverses direction of rays	Always erect Always virtual Always same size
Convex	Minus	Always erect Always virtual Always minified
Concave	Plus	Depends upon location of object Relative to focal point and center of curvature

Table 22-1   Mirrors

Angular magnification is used
- With objects and images at infinity (telescopes):

$$M_{telescope} = D_{eyepiece}/D_{objective}$$

- when viewing with an eye (simple magnifiers):

$$M_{simple\ magnifier} = D/4 \text{ (assumes 25 cm reference distance)}$$

Axial Magnification

Axial magnification compares relative image size (depth) along the optical axis. It is used with indirect ophthalmoscopy to determine image height or depth:

$$M_{Axial} = (\text{Transverse Magnification})^2$$

SPHERICAL EQUIVALENT

$$\text{Spherical equivalent} = \text{sphere} + \tfrac{1}{2} \text{ cylinder}$$

TRANSPOSITION OF CYLINDERS

New sphere = old sphere + old cylinder

New cylinder = old cylinder, but with opposite sign

New axis = old axis changed by 90°

VERTEX DISTANCE

Use the far point concept to
- Locate the focal point of the current lens.
- Determine the distance of the new lens to the far point of the eye. This is the focal length of the new lens.

- Take the reciprocal of the distance to determine the dioptric power of the lens.

Note: Vertex distance conversion is important for powers above ±5 D.

INTRAOCULAR LENS (IOL) CALCULATIONS

Saunders-Retzlaff-Kraff (SRK) Power for Emmetropia

$$P = A - 0.9 \text{ axial length} - 2.5 \text{ average K},$$

where A = the lens constant, supplied by the manufacturer, and K = keratometry reading.
- For each diopter of desired myopia in the spectacle plane, add between 1.25 and 1.5 D of IOL power.
- For each diopter of desired hyperopia in the spectacle plane, subtract between 1.25 and 1.5 D of IOL power.

MIRRORS

See Table 22-1.
- The central ray passes through the center of curvature (C).
- Use vergence formula (U + D = V) to locate images formed by mirrors.
- The reflecting power of a spherical mirror is

$$D_{reflecting} = 1/f = 1/(r/2) = 2/r,$$

where f = focal length in meters and r = radius of curvature in meters.

PATHOLOGY

MORTON E. SMITH

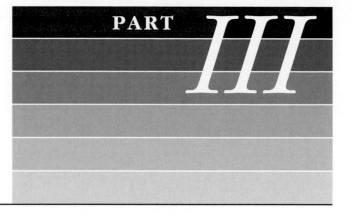

PART III

CHAPTER 23

Pathology

MELANOMAS AND LESIONS THAT SIMULATE MELANOMAS

Melanomas

Most pigmented tumors of the iris do not grow or grow at such a slow rate that they seldom jeopardize the patient's eye and certainly do not jeopardize the patient's life because they seldom metastasize to a distant site. These are nevi or low-grade, nonaggressive spindle cell melanomas. Clinically, these lesions are usually well demarcated, flat, and devoid of vessels. The more aggressive iris tumor is often a multicystic ("tapioca pudding") vascular lesion with ill-defined edges.

Histopathologic examination of most of these iris tumors shows cohesive fascicles of cells with spindle-shaped nuclei and ill-defined cytoplasmic borders. It appears that the cytoplasm of one cell blends imperceptibly into the cytoplasm of the adjacent cell. The nuclei are seldom nucleolated, and mitoses are rare (Figs. 23-1 and 23-2). These spindle cell melanomas differ from the more aggressive tumors, which are epithelioid melanomas. The latter are characterized by cells with large polygonal or round nuclei with prominent nucleoli, coarse clumping of chromatin, abundant eosinophilic cytoplasm, and well-defined cytoplasmic borders (Figs. 23-1 and 23-3). The occurrence of mitotic figures can range from rare to frequent.

Ciliary body and choroidal melanomas are more aggressive than the melanomas of the iris and often do metastasize, especially to the liver. The usual growth pattern is that of an elliptical-shaped tumor, which grows toward the vitreous (Fig. 23-4), and when the tumor

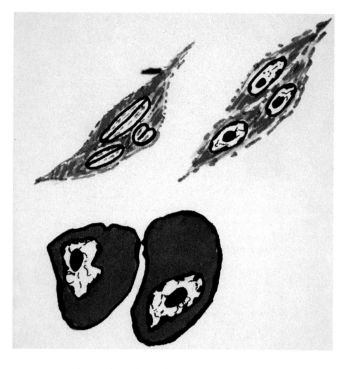

Fig. 23-1   In spindle A melanoma cells *(upper left)*, the nucleus is often grooved. In spindle B melanoma cells *(upper right)*, the spindle cell nucleus usually has a discernible nucleolus. In epithelioid melanoma cells *(lower half)*, the cytoplasmic border is discernible; there is abundant eosinophilic cytoplasm and a large nucleolated nucleus.

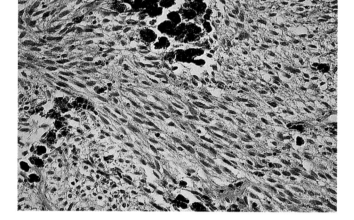

Fig. 23-2   Densely packed spindle A and B melanoma cells.

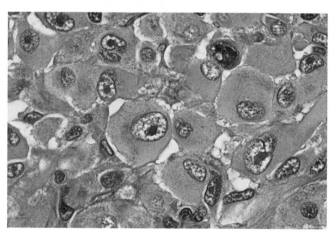

Fig. 23-3   Epithelioid melanoma cells.

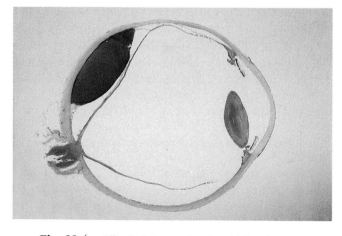

Fig. 23-4   Elliptical shape of a choroidal melanoma.

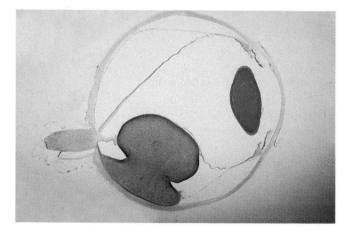

Fig. 23-5   The melanoma has broken through Bruch's membrane to assume the "mushroom" shape.

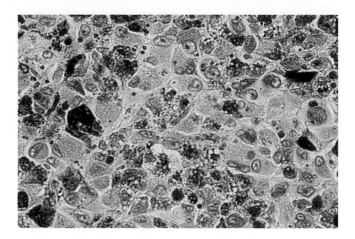

Fig. 23-6   Epithelioid melanoma cells.

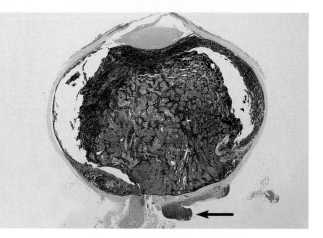

Fig. 23-8   The large melanoma fills the eye. Note the extrascleral extension *(arrow)*.

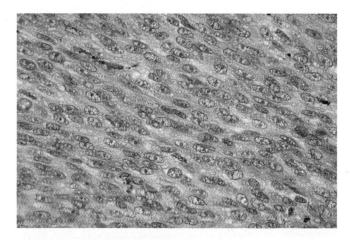

Fig. 23-7   Spindle B melanoma cells.

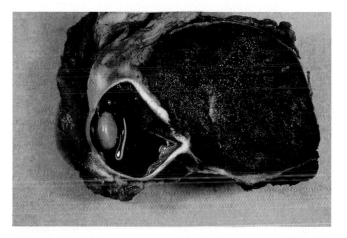

Fig. 23-9   Massive extrascleral extension.

Box 23-1   Characteristics of Melanomas That Predict Prognosis

1. Cell type: Epithelioid melanomas have a worse prognosis than spindle cell melanomas (Figs. 23-6 and 23-7).
2. Size: Large tumors have a worse prognosis than smaller tumors (Fig. 23-8).
3. Necrosis.
4. Number of mitoses.
5. Extrascleral extension (Fig. 23-9).
6. Location: Ciliary body melanomas and peripapillary melanomas have a worse prognosis.
7. Vascular pattern.

---

breaks through Bruch's membrane, it assumes a "mushroom" shape (Fig. 23-5).

There are several histopathologic features of ciliary body and choroidal melanomas that predict prognosis for survival (Box 23-1 and Figs. 23-6 to 23-9).

Lesions That Simulate Intraocular Melanomas

Intraocular melanomas may be clinically confused with subretinal hemorrhage, inflammatory lesions, cavernous hemangiomas, metastatic carcinoma, and lymphoma. The most common primary carcinomas that metastasize to the uveal tract (usually the choroid) are breast in woman and lung in men. These metastatic carcinomas usually are relatively flat (compared to the mushroom configuration of melanoma) and are often multifocal as well as bilateral (Fig. 23-10).

RETINOBLASTOMA

The characteristic clinical manifestation of retinoblastoma is leukocoria (Fig. 23-11). Histopathologically, the tumor arises from the retina and is composed of densely packed cells with basophilic staining nuclei and scant cytoplasm (Figs. 23-12 and 23-13). These tumor cells

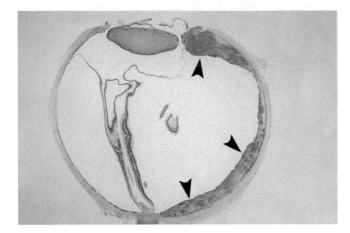

Fig. 23-10   The right half of the choroids is thickened by a flat, diffuse metastatic carcinoma *(arrowheads)*.

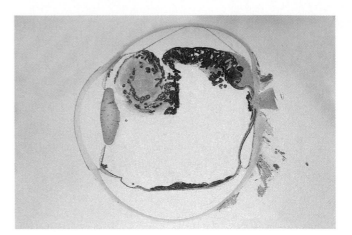

Fig. 23-12   Retinoblastoma. Blue tumor and pink necrosis.

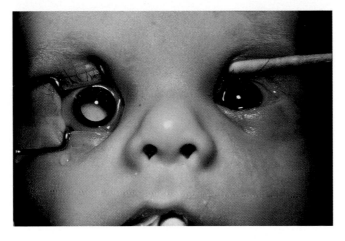

Fig. 23-11   Right eye with leukocoria in retinoblastoma.

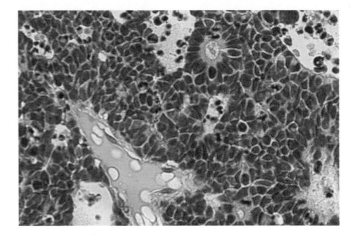

Fig. 23-13   Retinoblastoma. Densely packed cells with blue nuclei and scant cytoplasm.

form islands within pools of pink necrosis (Fig. 23-14). Mitosis is frequently seen (Fig. 23-15). The Flexner-Wintersteiner rosette consists of a single ring of cells around an empty lumen (Fig. 23-16). The pseudorosette is a cluster of retinoblastoma cells around a central blood vessel (Fig. 23-17). Scattered flecks of calcium are frequently seen.

Prognosis is predicted by the extent of the tumor. Extension of tumor into the optic nerve, especially at the surgical margin of the nerve, and massive invasion into the choroid indicate a poor prognosis (Fig. 23-18).

ADNEXAL LESIONS

Lids

Basal cell carcinoma is the most common neoplasm of the skin of the lids, and the skin of the lids (especially the lower lid) is one of the most common sites for basal cell

carcinoma. Histopathologic examination shows islands of cells arising from the surface epithelium and extending into the subepithelial stroma. The nuclei are round and oval with scant cytoplasm, and there is palisading ("picket fence") of the cells at the periphery of the islands (Fig. 23-19). Basal cell carcinoma rarely metastasizes to a distant site but can invade locally. The morphea type (Fig. 23-20) is considered to be a more aggressive type of basal cell carcinoma.

Sebaceous gland carcinoma may present as a recurrent chalazion, a mass, or chronic unilateral blepharoconjunctivitis. The loss of cilia is a characteristic clinical finding in this entity. Histopathologically, the tumor is composed of cells with basophilic nuclei and lipid vacuoles within most of the cells (Fig. 23-21). Intraepithelial spread of the tumor along the conjunctiva is referred to as pagetoid spread (Fig. 23-22).

Differentiating (microscopically) sebaceous gland carcinoma from a chalazion is not difficult. A chalazion is

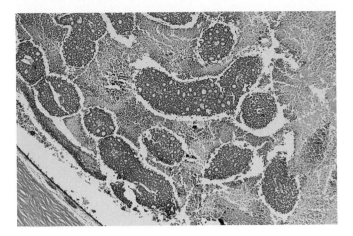

Fig. 23-14   Retinoblastoma: "islands of blue tumor in a sea of pink necrosis."

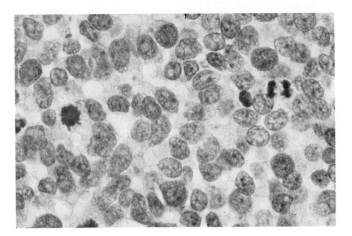

Fig. 23-15   Mitotic figures are often seen in retinoblastoma.

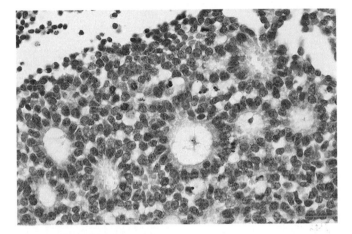

Fig. 23-16   A single ring of retinoblastoma cells around a clear lumen is the Flexner-Wintersteiner rosette.

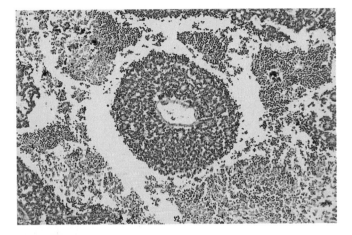

Fig. 23-17   A cluster of retinoblastoma cells around a blood vessel is referred to as a pseudorosette.

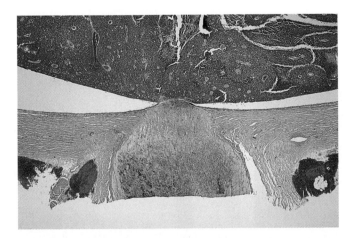

Fig. 23-18   The blue retinoblastoma cells can be seen in the optic nerve.

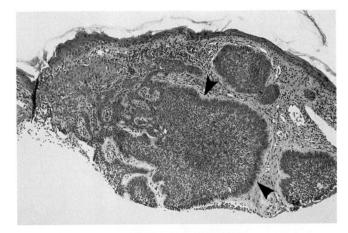

Fig. 23-19   Basal cell carcinoma. Note the characteristic palisading of cells around the periphery of each island of tumor cells *(arrowheads).*

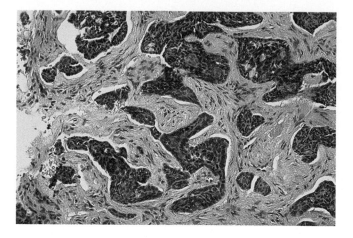

Fig. 23-20   Morpheaform basal cell is the more aggressive form.

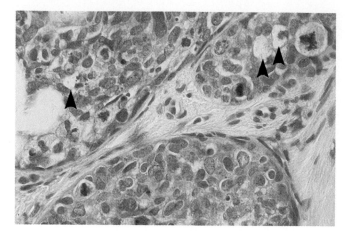

Fig. 23-21   Sebaceous gland carcinoma. Note the clear lipid vacuoles *(arrowheads)*.

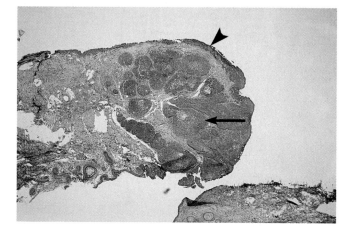

Fig. 23-22   Sebaceous gland carcinoma. Note the pagetoid spread along the conjunctiva *(arrowhead)*. The main part of the tumor is deeper in the stroma *(arrow)*.

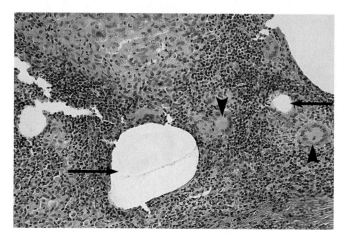

Fig. 23-23   Chalazion. Note the clear lipid vacuoles *(arrows)* and the granulomatous inflammation with giant cells *(arrowheads)*.

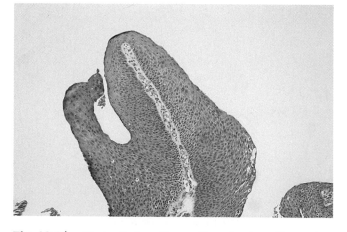

Fig. 23-24   Conjuctival papilloma. Note the fingerlike projections of acanthotic epithelium with a fibrovascular core.

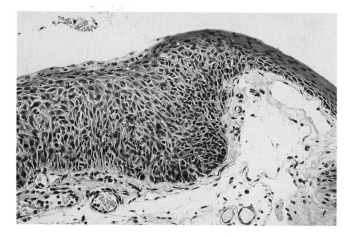

Fig. 23-25   CIN. Note the abrupt change from normal epithelium *(right)* to thickened epithelium *(left)*.

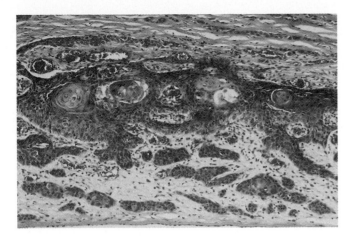

Fig. 23-26   Squamous cell carcinoma of the conjunctiva has spread into the cornea.

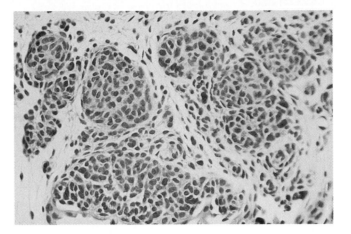

Fig. 23-27   Conjunctival nevus. Note the nests of blue nuclei.

merely a classical example of lipogranulomatous inflammation (Fig. 23-23).

Other lid neoplasms include squamous cell carcinoma, keratoacanthoma, and melanoma. Common benign lesions include seborrheic keratosis and benign cysts.

Conjunctiva

Epithelial tumors   Papillomas appear clinically as pink vascular "mulberry" lesions. Histopathologically, these are fingerlike projections of thickened (acanthotic) epithelium with a central fibrovascular core (Fig. 23-24).

Dysplasia and carcinoma-in-situ (conjunctival intraepithelial neoplasia [CIN]) have a leukoplakia type of growth at the limbus and across the cornea. Histopathologically, the lesion shows varying degrees of pleomorphism throughout the thickened epithelium, but the basement membrane remains intact (Fig. 23-25).

Squamous cell carcinoma shows a greater degree of cytologic pleomorphism than CIN and invades through the basement membrane into the underlying tissue (Fig. 23-26).

Melanocytic tumors of the conjunctiva   Nevi are common, and most remain stationary throughout life. Excisional biopsy is done for atypical lesions, for lesions that change in size and/or appearance, and for cosmesis. Histopathologic examination shows nests (Fig. 23-27) of cells with basophilic nuclei, which are round, oval, and pear-shaped. The cytoplasmic borders are indistinguishable. The nuclei often show clear pseudovacuoles. Epithelial inclusion cysts are commonly found among the nests of nevus cells (Fig. 23-28).

Primary acquired melanosis (PAM) characteristically occurs in adult life in persons of fair complexion. It is unilateral and initially starts as a superficial "dusting" of

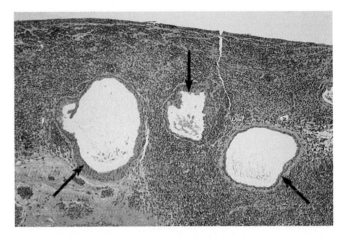

Fig. 23-28   Conjunctival nevus. Epithelial microcysts are common in benign nevi *(arrows)*.

melanin pigment. It tends to wax and wane but may give rise to melanoma. Histopathologically, there is an increased number of melanocytes along the basal layer of epithelial cells, and these may show varying degrees of atypia (Fig. 23-29).

Melanoma of the conjunctiva is rare. It may arise from a preexisting nevus, from PAM, or de novo. Histopathologically, the cells are spindle or epithelioid or both. There is discohesiveness and pleomorphism (Fig. 23-30). Metastasis is usually regional to the preauricular, submandibular, or anterior cervical lymph nodes.

Lymphoma   The clinical appearance of lymphoma of the conjunctiva is the pink "salmon patch." Histologically, these lesions range from benign lymphoid hyperplasia (with germinal centers and small round mature lymphocyte) to large, irregular lymphocytes with coarse clumping of chromatin and mitotic figures. The intermediate pattern is that of a low-grade lymphoma ("MALT," i.e., mucosa-associated lymphoid tumor).

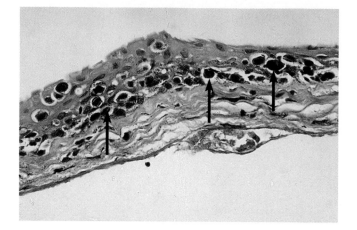

Fig. 23-29   Primary acquired melanosis. Note the pigmented cells along the basal layer of the epithelium *(arrows).*

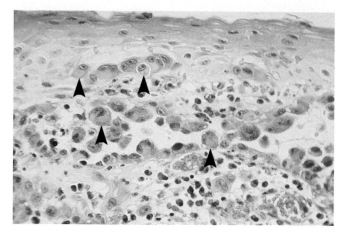

Fig. 23-30   Melanoma of the conjunctiva. Note the discohesive epithelioid cells *(arrowheads).*

Table 23-1   Other conjunctival lesions

Lesion	Histopathologic characteristics
Dermoid	Skin
Dermolipoma	Skin and adipose tissue
Pinguecula	Elastotic degeneration
Pterygium	Elastotic degeneration and hypervascularity
Cyst	Lining of cyst is conjunctival epithelium
Ocular cicatricial pemphigoid	Subepithelial bullae and immunoglobulin deposition in basement membrane

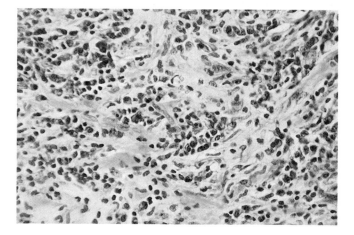

Fig. 23-31   Idiopathic orbital inflammation ("inflammatory pseudotumors"). There are many different inflammatory cells as well as fibroconnective tissue.

Other conjunctival lesions   Other conjunctival lesions are listed in Table 23-1.

Orbit

Grave's ophthalmopathy   Although Grave's ophthalmopathy is the most common cause of orbital disease, there is seldom a need for tissue biopsy. In the rare cases for which a tissue biopsy is available, the microscopic examination reveals lymphocytes and mast cells between the fibers of the extraocular muscles.

Idiopathic orbital inflammation ("inflammatory pseudotumor")   Although most patients with this condition do not have systemic disease, occasionally there is an associated collagen-vascular disease such as Wegener's granulomatosis. Histopathologic examination shows infiltration of the orbital tissues by chronic inflammatory cells including lymphocytes, plasma cells, eosinophiles,

epithelioid cells, and variable degrees of fibroconnective tissue (Fig. 23-31).

Vascular and vascular-like tumors   Cavernous hemangiomas usually occur in young adults, and they characteristically appear as round or oval well-demarcated solid tumors in the muscle cone when viewed by magnetic resonance imaging or computed tomography (Fig. 23-32). Histopathologically, there are large vascular spaces filled with erythrocytes, separated by thick and thin fibrous septa (Fig. 23-33).

Capillary hemangiomas typically appear in the first year of life. They may be well demarcated or diffusely spread in the lids, conjunctiva, and orbit. Histopathologically, there are small vascular spaces separated by thin hypercellular septa (Fig. 23-34).

Histopathologic examination of lymphangiomas shows spaces filled with blood and protein, and there are often aggregations of lymphocytes in the fibrous septa.

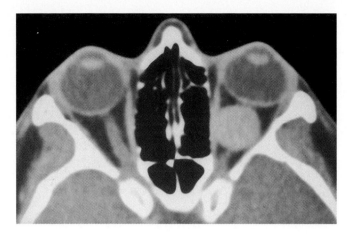

Fig. 23-32   A cavernous hemangioma is a well-demarcated round lesion in the muscle cone.

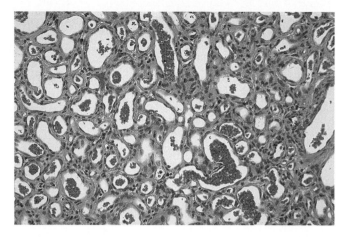

Fig. 23-34   Capillary hemangioma: small blood-filled spaces separated by cellular septa.

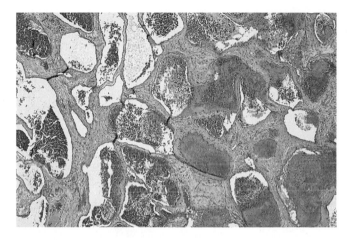

Fig. 23-33   Cavernous hemangioma: large blood-filled spaces separated by fibrous septa.

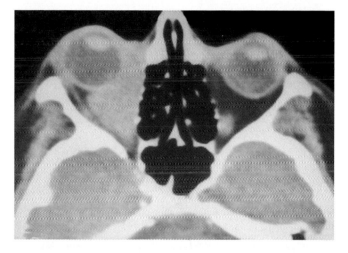

Fig. 23-35   Lymphomas "mold" to globe and orbital wall

Lymphomas   Lymphomas characteristically appear as a "molded" tumor in the orbit; i.e., the tumor molds itself against the globe and/or orbital walls (Fig. 23-35). Histopathologically, these tumors can range from benign lymphoid hyperplasia to low-grade lymphomas to high-grade lymphomas (Fig. 23-36).

Lacrimal gland tumors   Most of the reasons for enlargement of the lacrimal gland are infiltrations rather than intrinsic neoplasms, e.g., sarcoid, lymphoma, dacryadenitis, or pseudotumor. Of the intrinsic neoplasms, pleomorphic adenoma (also known as benign mixed tumor of the lacrimal gland) is the most common. Histopathologic examination shows epithelial and mesenchymal elements (Fig. 23-37). The most common malignant neoplasm is the adenoid cystic carcinoma, which has been described as a "Swiss cheese" pattern when seen under the microscope because of the "holes" in the clusters of malignant cells (Fig. 23-38).

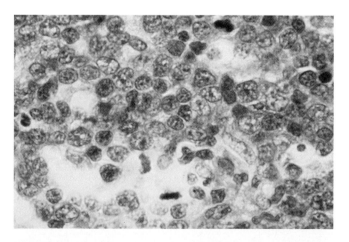

Fig. 23-36   Lymphoma: round nuclei with scant cytoplasm. Note the irregular and angulated nuclear borders and coarse clumping of chromatin.

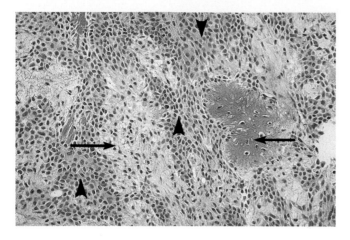

Fig. 23-37 Pleomorphic adenoma (benign mixed cell tumor). Note epithelial cells *(arrowheads)* as well as mesenchymal elements *(arrows)*.

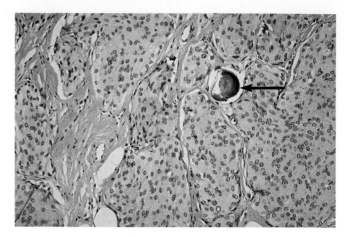

Fig. 23-40 Meningioma: nests of pale oval nuclei, pink cytoplasm, and a psammoma body *(arrow)*.

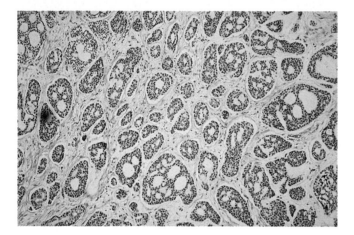

Fig. 23-38 Adenoid cystic carcinoma. Note that the tumor cells form a "Swiss cheese" pattern.

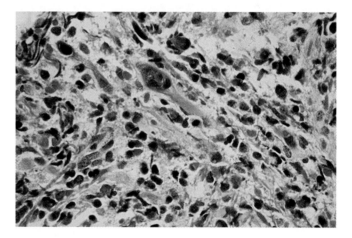

Fig. 23-41 Rhabdomyosarcoma: hyperchromatic irregular nuclei with pink cytoplasm.

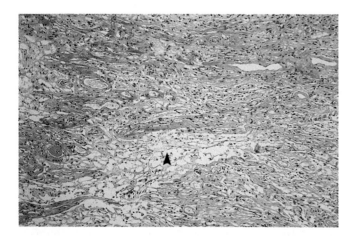

Fig. 23-39 Optic nerve glioma. Note the myxoid background *(arrowhead)*.

Optic nerve glioma and perioptic meningioma Histopathologically, a glioma is characterized by overgrowth of glial cells against a myxoid (loose network) background (Fig. 23-39). A meningioma has whorls of pale-staining cells, often with psammoma bodies present (Fig. 23-40).

Rhabdomyosarcoma Rhabdomyosarcoma is a rare tumor but is the most common orbital malignancy in children (average age 7 years). Histopathologically, the hyperchromatic irregular nuclei show marked pleomorphism with pink cytoplasm in the form of "balls" and "ribbons" (Fig. 23-41).

Dermoid cysts Dermoid cysts are lined by squamous epithelium and filled with keratin.

Other rare diseases of the orbit Other rare diseases of the orbit are listed in Box 23-2.

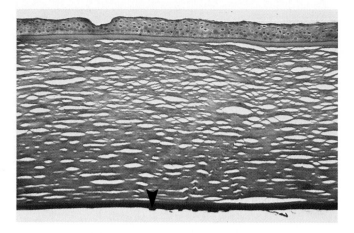

Fig. 23-42   Fuch's dystrophy. Note the absence of endothelial cells and the presence of guttata *(arrowhead)*.

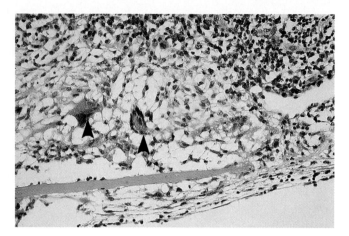

Fig. 23-43   Herpes simplex keratitis. The stroma is infiltrated by inflammatory cells. Note the giant cells *(arrowheads)* near Descemet's membrane.

Box 23-2   Other Rare Diseases of the Orbit

Neurofibroma	Alveolar soft part sarcoma
Neurilemmoma	Juvenile xanthogranuloma
Fibrous histiocytoma	Langerhans cell tumors
Hemangiopericytoma	Sinus histiocytosis
Granular cell tumor	

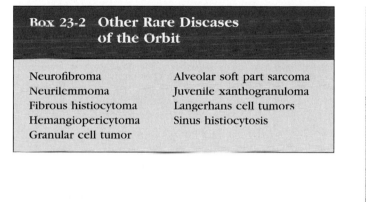

CORNEA AND SCLERA

Endothelial Decompensation

A common histopathologic diagnosis of a corneal "button" (host cornea) from a corneal transplant procedure is endothelial decompensation, either pseudophakic bullous keratopathy or Fuch's dystrophy. The characteristic histopathologic feature is seen at the level of endothelium and Descemet's membrane. Endothelial cells are sparse and in Fuch's dystrophy there are excrescences (guttata) (Fig. 23-42); the secondary changes in the epithelium include edema of the basal layer and bullae.

Herpes Simplex Keratitis

Histopathologic examination shows patchy or complete loss of Bowman's layer, chronic inflammatory cell infiltration in the stroma, vascularization of the stroma, and often a granulomatous inflammation in or near Descemet's membrane (Fig. 23-43).

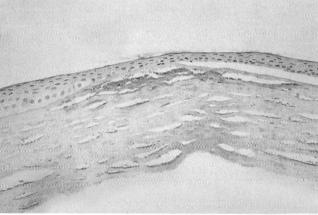

Fig. 23-44   Macular dystrophy. The Alcian blue stain is positive for acid mucopolysaccharide.

Hereditary Stromal Dystrophies

In macular dystrophy an accumulation of acid mucopolysaccharide is seen. The Alcian blue stain is positive (Fig. 23-44).

With granular dystrophy, a hyaline degeneration is seen, which stains positively with Masson trichrome stain (Fig. 23-45).

In lattice dystrophy amyloid deposition, which stains positively with Congo red, is present (Fig. 23-46).

Keratitis

Nonulcerative   Histopathologically, interstitial keratitis due to congenital syphilis is characterized by stromal scarring and vascularization, which are most prominent in the posterior stroma.

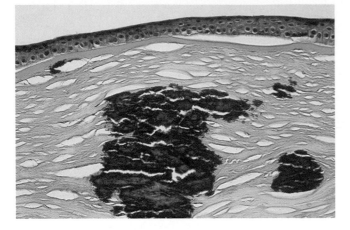

Fig. 23-45 Granular dystrophy. The mason trichrome stain is positive (red) for hyaline deposition.

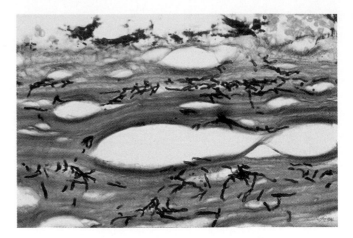

Fig. 23-47 Fungi are easily seen with Gomori methenamine silver (GMS) stain.

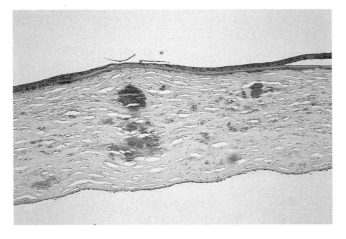

Fig. 23-46 Lattice dystrophy. The Congo red stain (orange) is positive for amyloid.

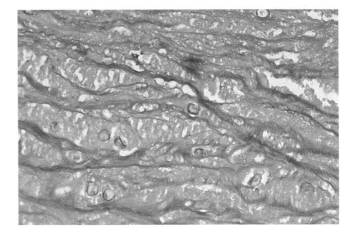

Fig. 23-48 Acanthamoebae are circular and seen with stains (periodic acid-Schiff, GMS, or calcofluor white).

Ulcerative keratitis Results of histopathologic examination in patients with Mooren's and Terrien's keratitis are nonspecific, showing only chronic inflammation and varying degrees of vascularization.

Acute and chronic inflammatory cell infiltration and necrosis are the hallmarks of bacterial and fungal keratitis. Special stains are used to identify the incriminating organism (Fig. 23-47). Acanthamoebae have gained notoriety in the past two decades, and special stains facilitate their identification (Fig. 23-48). With infectious crystalline keratopathy colonies of bacteria in the mid stroma, often with an overlying intact epithelium, are seen.

The sequelae of chronic corneal disease include the following:

• Stromal fibrosis shows loss of the clefts.
• Band keratopathy is calcification of Bowman's layer.

• Pannus is a growth under the epithelium; it can be vascular, fibrotic, inflammatory, or a combination of all of these.

Keratoconus

Keratoconus is another common reason for corneal transplant surgery. Histopathologic examination shows central thinning and fibrosis and small breaks in Bowman's layer (Fig. 23-49).

Scleritis

With scleritis varying degrees of inflammation and necrosis are present. This is usually granulomatous in nature, and seldom is a microorganism identified.

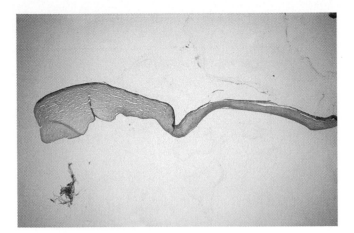

Fig. 23-49 Keratoconus. The central cornea is thinner than the periphery.

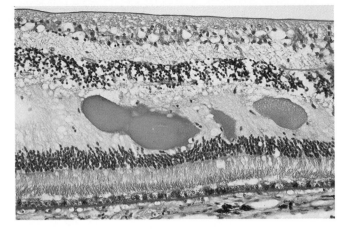

Fig. 23-51 In diabetes, "pockets" of lipoproteinaceous exudates are seen in the deeper layer of the retina.

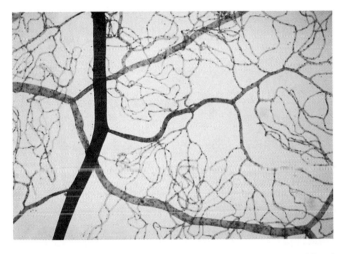

Fig. 23-50 Typsin digestion preparation of retinal blood vessels.

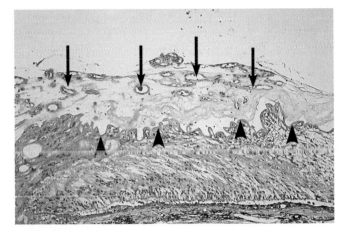

Fig. 23-52 A sheet of neovascular tissue *(arrows)* lies internal to the wrinkled internal limiting membrane of the retina *(arrowheads)*.

RETINA AND OPTIC NERVE

Diabetes

Early histopathologic changes are best seen by studying the capillaries after trypsin digestion (Fig. 23-50). The changes include thickening of the basement membrane, selective loss of the intramural pericytes, microaneurysm formation, and capillary drop out. These changes are followed by lipoproteinaceous exudates and hemorrhages in the mid and deep layers of the neurosensory retina (Fig. 23-51). Neovascularization is then seen on the inner surface of the retina (Fig. 23-52).

The iris eventually shows surface neovascularization (rubeosis) and peripheral anterior synechiae, which close the angle (Fig. 23-53). Vacuolization of the iris pigment epithelium is seen when the patient's blood glucose level is elevated at the time of the enucleation (clinical or autopsy) (Fig. 23-54).

Hypertension and Vascular Occlusive Disease

Intraretinal hemorrhage is the hallmark of these diseases (Fig. 23-55). With central retinal vein occlusion, as the blood resorbs, the inner two-thirds of the retina shows architectural disarray and cystoid degeneration (Fig. 23-56). Lipoproteinaceous exudates and neovascularization similar to those seen with diabetes are also present.

The histopathologic correlate of ophthalmoscopic cotton-wool spots is the cytoid body, which is a micro-

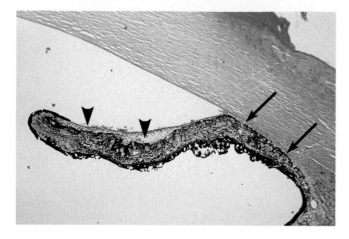

Fig. 23-53   Diabetes. Note the neovascularization on the anterior surface of the iris *(arrowheads)*. The angle is closed by peripheral anterior synechiae *(arrows)*.

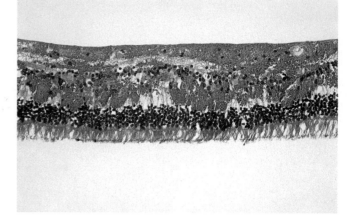

Fig. 23-55   Diffuse intraretinal hemorrhage occupies the inner two-thirds of the retina.

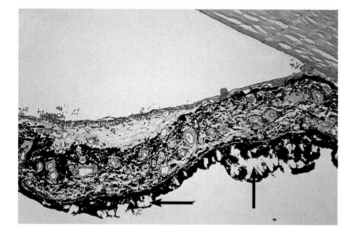

Fig. 23-54   Diabetes. Note the vacuolization of the iris pigment epithelium *(arrows)*.

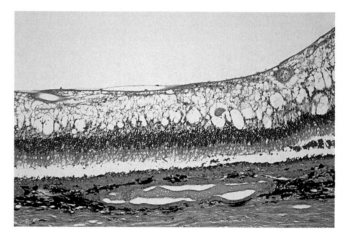

Fig. 23-56   There is diffuse cystoid degeneration of the inner two-thirds of the retina.

infarct in the nerve fiber layer. These cytoid bodies are ganglion cell axons, which are swollen by stagnant axoplasm (Fig. 23-57).

Age-Related Macular Degeneration (ARMD)
(Figs. 23-58 and 23-59)

The histopathologic features of ARMD include the following:

1. Thickening and calcification of Bruch's membrane
2. Drusen
3. Deterioration of retinal pigment epithelium (RPE) cells
4. Breaks in Bruch's membrane
5. Neovascular membrane between RPE and Bruch's membrane

OPTIC NERVE

Papilledema, Inflammation, Infarct, Atrophy

In papilledema, there is elevation of the nerve head toward the vitreous as well as lateral displacement of the neurosensory elements of the retina (Fig. 23-60). Chronic inflammatory cell infiltration characterizes papillitis. With temporal arteritis, it is not, of course, the infarcted nerve that is submitted to the pathology laboratory but a biopsy specimen from a temporal artery. The characteristic histopathologic features for a positive diagnosis of temporal arteritis include a narrowed lumen and a granulomatous inflammation of the walls of the vessel. Giant cells may or may not be seen (Fig. 23-61).

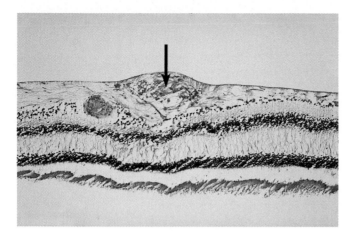

Fig. 23-57 Cytoid body *(arrow)* is a microinfarct in the nerve fiber layer of the retina and corresponds to the cotton-wool spot seen with the ophthalmoscope.

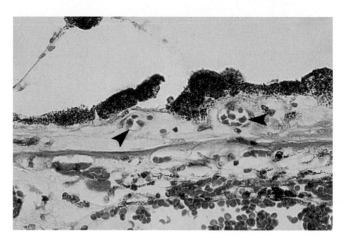

Fig. 23-59 Age-related macular degeneration. Note the neovascular membrane *(arrowheads)* between RPE and Bruch's membrane.

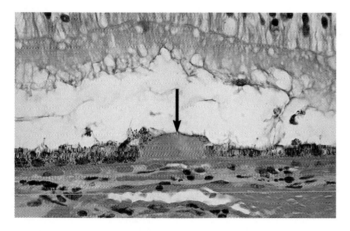

Fig. 23-58 A druse *(arrow)* rests on Bruch's membrane.

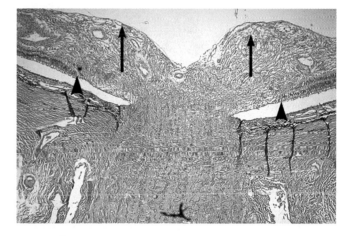

Fig. 23-60 Papilledema. Note the elevation of the nerve head toward the vitreous *(arrows)* and the lateral displacement of the neurosensory retina *(arrowheads)*.

Neoplasms

The two most frequent neoplasms associated with the optic nerve are gliomas and optic nerve sheath meningiomas (see "Orbit," discussed previously in this chapter).

INFLAMMATION AND INFECTIONS

Postoperative Endophthalmitis

Postoperative endophthalmitis is characterized by massive infiltration throughout the vitreous, retina, and choroid by polymorphonuclear leukocytes with varying degrees of tissue necrosis (Fig. 23-62). These infiltrations are usually bacterial (less frequently fungal) and are seen with appropriate stains, such as tissue Gram stain for bacteria and silver stain for fungi.

Infectious Retinitis and Uveitis

Herpes zoster is characterized by lymphocytes and plasma cells infiltrating the cornea and iris and around the nerves in the sclera (perineural).

Cytomegalovirus infection, especially in the retina, has been described as an "owl's eye" because of the prominent intranuclear inclusion body surrounded by a clear halo (Fig. 23-63).

Toxoplasmosis affects the retina with a secondary lymphocyte infiltration in the choroid and vitreous. The *Toxoplasma* cysts may be seen within the necrotic retina (Fig. 23-64).

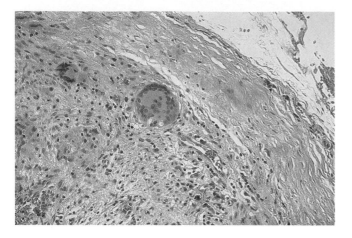

Fig. 23-61   Temporal arteritis. There is a granulomatous inflammation of the wall of the artery. Note the giant cell in the *center* of the figure.

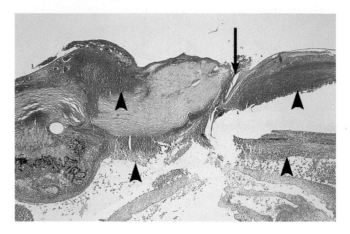

Fig. 23-62   Endophthalmitis after corneal transplant surgery. All tissues are infiltrated by acute inflammatory cells *(arrowheads).* Note the corneal wound *(arrow).*

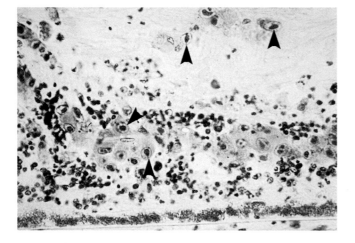

Fig. 23-63   *Cytomegalovirus* retinitis. The prominent intranuclear inclusion body with a clear "halo" produces the "owl's eye" appearance *(arrowheads).*

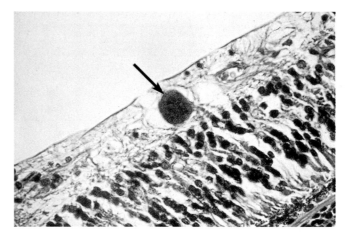

Fig. 23-64   Toxoplasmosis. The cyst is in the nerve fiber layer of the retina *(arrow).*

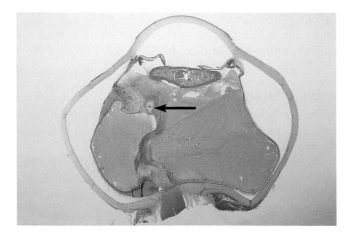

Fig. 23-65   *Toxocara canis* endophthalmitis. The vitreous abscess contains eosinophiles *(arrow).*

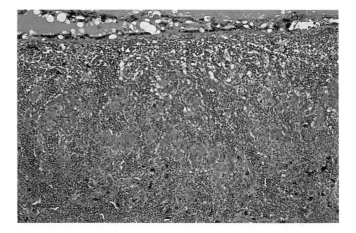

Fig. 23-66   Sympathetic ophthalmia. The choroid is infiltrated by lymphocytes *(dark cells)* and aggregates of epithelioid cells *(lighter areas).*

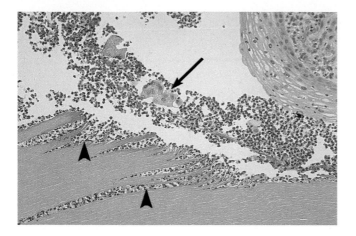

Fig. 23-67 Phacoantigenic inflammation. Acute inflammatory cells infiltrate the lens *(arrowheads)*, and there is a surrounding granulomatous inflammation, including giant cells *(arrows)*.

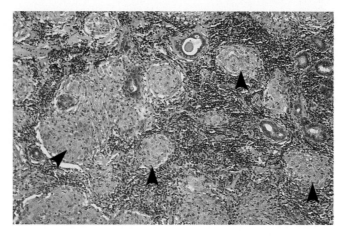

Fig. 23-68 Sarcoidosis. Note the tubercles of granulomatous inflammation *(arrowheads)*.

The characteristic finding in patients with *Toxocara canis* endophthalmitis is the eosinophilic abscess in the vitreous (Fig. 23-65). The organism is seldom found.

Noninfectious Inflammatory Diseases

Sympathetic ophthalmia is a rare bilateral disease, which follows a penetrating injury of one eye. The histopathologic appearance is characteristic and includes diffuse granulomatous uveitis with lymphocytes and scattered focal aggregations of epithelioid cells and giant cells (Fig. 23-66). There is a relative sparing of the choriocapillaris, and plasma cells are infrequent. Pigment phagocytosis is seen in the cytoplasm of the epithelioid cells. Eosinophils are often seen, and clusters of epithelioid cells along Bruch's membrane are known as Dalen-Fuchs nodules.

Phacoantigenic ("phacoanaphylaxis") inflammation follows rupture of the lens capsule with infiltration of polymorphonuclear leukocytes into the lens and a surrounding zone of granulomatous inflammation (Fig. 23-67).

Sarcoidosis may affect the lids, conjunctiva, uvea, retina, optic nerve, lacrimal gland, and orbit. The most common site for biopsy is the granulomatous nodule in the palpebral conjunctiva. The characteristic histopathologic appearance is the noncaseating tubercle of epithelioid cells and giant cells surrounded by lymphocytes (Fig. 23-68).

TRAUMA

With penetrating and perforating injuries to the globe varying degrees of distortion and repair (scar formation)

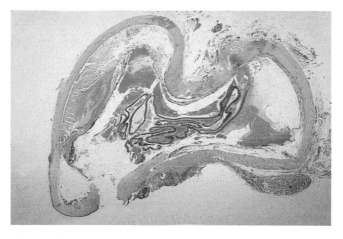

Fig. 23-69 Ruptured globe with massive intraocular hemorrhage.

will be seen, ranging from scars from simple wound healing of the cornea to "rupture of the globe with massive intraocular hemorrhage" (Fig. 23-69). If the globe rupture progresses to phthisis, the characteristic histopathologic findings are severe architectural distortion, atrophy, and ossification of the RPE (Fig. 23-70).

Epithelial down-growth may occur through a poorly apposed traumatic or surgical wound (Fig. 23-71).

Nonpenetrating (blunt) trauma often results in a postcontusion angle recession. The iris root inserts far posterior to the scleral spur because of the tear in the face of the ciliary body (Fig. 23-72).

Severe blunt trauma involving the retina will often resemble retinitis pigmentosa, in which the pigment from the retinal pigment epithelial layer migrates into the atrophic neurosensory retina.

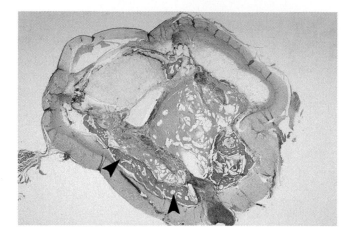

Fig. 23-70   Atrophia bulbi ("phthisis bulbi"). Note the ossification of the RPE *(arrowheads)*.

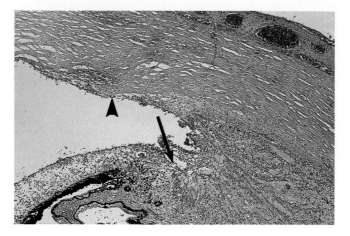

Fig. 23-72   Postcontusion angle recession. The iris root is retrodisplaced *(arrow);* the normal position is at the scleral spur *(arrowhead).*

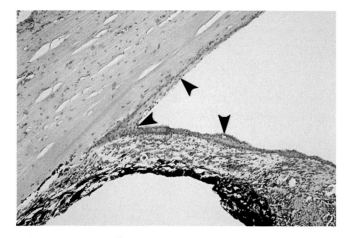

Fig. 23-71   Epithelium lines the posterior surface of the cornea, the angle, and the anterior surface of the iris *(arrowheads).*

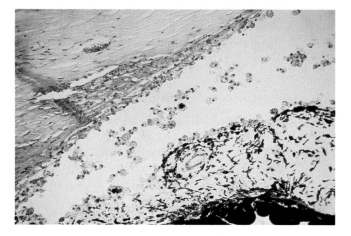

Fig. 23-73   Phacolytic glaucoma. Lens-laden macrophages fill the anterior chamber and "clog" the trabecular meshwork.

GLAUCOMA

Specimens of globes with primary open angle glaucoma and primary angle closure glaucoma seldom reach the pathology laboratory.

Secondary glaucomas do provide the specimens that may eventually reach pathology laboratories. These secondary glaucomas can be divided into two groups: open angle and closed angle.

Secondary Open Angle Glaucoma

In these globes, the angle is anatomically open, but there are cells or debris that clog the trabecular meshwork.

Phacolytic glaucoma is characterized by large lens-laden macrophages that have ingested the liquified cortical lens material leaking through the intact capsule of a hypermature cataract (Fig. 23-73).

In erythrocyte-induced glaucoma, the trabecular meshwork is clogged with erythrocytes, "ghost" erythrocytes, hemosiderin-laden macrophages, or a combination of all three (Fig. 23-74).

Secondary Closed Angle Glaucoma (Peripheral Anterior Synechiae)

Most secondary closed angle glaucomas (Fig. 23-75) can be grouped into seven broad categories as follows:
  1. Forward displacement of iris-lens diaphragm, e.g., intraocular tumor

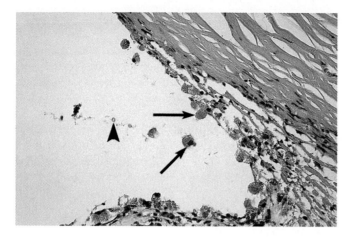

Fig. 23-74 Hemosiderin-laden macrophages *(arrows)* and "ghost" erythrocytes fill the anterior chamber and "clog" the trabecular meshwork.

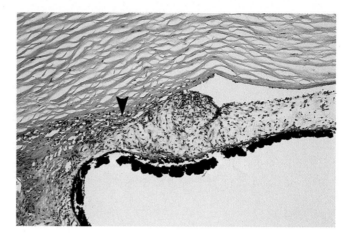

Fig. 23-75 Peripheral anterior synechiae occlude the angle. The trabecular meshwork is at the *arrowhead.*

KEY FEATURES

Disease	Key histopathologic features
Melanoma	Spindle cells and epithelioid cells; choroidal "mushroom"
Metastatic carcinoma	Flat, diffuse growth in choroid
Retinoblastoma	Blue cells and pink necrosis and flecks of calcium
Basal cell carcinoma	Palisading at edge of islands of tumor
Sebaceous gland carcinoma	Lipid vacuoles in cells
CIN	Malignant squamous cells with intact basement membrane
Idiopathic orbital inflammation	Polymorphic inflammatory cells with fibroconnective tissue
Vascular tumors	Small lumens: capillary; large lumens: cavernous
Lymphomas, malignant	Large round cells with irregular edges and course clumping of nuclear chromatin
Pleomorphic adenoma	Epithelial elements and mesenchymal elements
Adenoid cystic carcinoma	"Swiss cheese" pattern
Rhabdomyosarcoma	Blue irregular nuclei with pink cytoplasm
Herpes simplex keratitis	Loss of Bowman's layer, stromal inflammation, and granulomatous inflammation near Descemet's membrane
Fuch's dystrophy	Loss of endothelial cells and guttata
Pseudophakic bullous keratopathy	Loss of endothelial cells, no guttata
Keratoconus	Central thinning and fibrosis and small disruptions of Bowman's layer
Diabetes	Intraretinal hemorrhage and exudates; neovascularization of retina and iris; "lacy" vacuolization of iris pigment epithelium
ARMD	Thickening and calcification of Bruch's membrane; drusen; disruption of RPE; neovascular membrane between RPE and Bruch's membrane
Sympathic uveitis	Diffuse granulomatous uveitis with lack of plasma cells
Phacoantigenic inflammation	Granulomatous inflammation surrounds a ruptured lens capsule
Phacolytic glaucoma	Lens laden macrophages in anterior chamber and trabecular meshwork
Postcontusion angle recession	Retrodisplacement of iris root

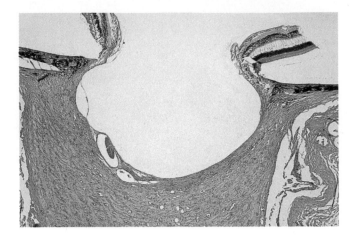

Fig. 23-76   Glaucomatous cupping of the disk.

2. Chronic iritis
3. Previous anterior segment surgery
4. Trauma; blunt and penetrating
5. Ice syndrome
6. Neovascularization of the iris and angle ("rubeosis"), e.g., central retinal vein occlusion or diabetes
7. Recurrent angle closure attacks

Optic Nerve and Retina

The changes in the optic nerve and retina include cupping (Fig. 23-76), gliosis, and thickening of the pial septa. Occasionally, Schnabel's cavernous atrophy is present, in which there is a demarcated area of "spongy" infarcted optic nerve tissue.

The retina shows atrophy and gliosis of the nerve fiber layer and loss of ganglion cells. The inner nuclear layer remains intact, in contrast to a central retinal vascular occlusion, in which there is destruction of the inner nuclear layer.

SUGGESTED READINGS

Apple D, Rapp M, editors: *Ocular pathology: clinical applications and self-assessment,* ed 4, St Louis, 1991, Mosby.

Eagle R: *Eye pathology, an atlas and basic text,* Philadelphia, 1999, WB Saunders.

Garner A, Klintworth G, editors: *Pathobiology of ocular disease,* New York, 1994, Dekker.

Sassani J, editor: *Ophthalmic pathology with clinical correlations,* Philadelphia, 1997, Lippincott-Raven.

Spencer W, editor: *Ophthalmic pathology, an atlas and textbook,* ed 4, Philadelphia, 1996, WB Saunders.

Yanoff M, Fine B: *Ocular pathology,* ed 4, St Louis, 1996, Mosby.

Index

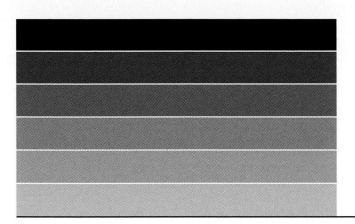

Page numbers followed by *f* indicate figures; page numbers followed by *t* indicate tables.